flexibility

flexibility

Alan Gordon

MQP

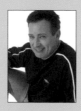

About the author

Alan Gordon began his career over thirty years ago at the Royal Air Force School of Physical Training. Since then he has worked as a professional exercise and nutritional consultant, with a client list that spans the worlds of both sport and media celebrities. He has a Masters Degree in Biomechanics and Applied Human Movement, an Honours degree in Nutrition, an Advanced Clinical Diploma in Stress Management, and is a highly advanced expert in improving strength, flexibility, and total body fitness. You can contact him via his website: www.alangordon-health.co.uk

Caution

If you suffer from any medical conditions or injuries, or are pregnant or undertaking an exercise program for the first time, consult your doctor and seek advice from a qualified fitness professional beforehand. This book is meant as guidance only, and if you feel any pain or discomfort while exercising you should stop immediately.

Picture Credits

p.12: © Rob Lewine/CORBIS; p.17: © Randy M. Ury/CORBIS; p.124: © Tim Pannell/CORBIS; p.130: © Stuart Hughes/CORBIS; p.132: © Lawrence Manning/CORBIS; p.136: © Tom Stewart/CORBIS; p.138: © Ed Bock/CORBIS; p.140: © Cory Sorensen/CORBIS; p.142: © Hughes Martin/CORBIS; p.146: © Chuck Savage/CORBIS; p.148: © Superstock Photo Library.

Published by MQ Publications Limited

12 The Ivories
6–8 Northampton Street
London N1 2HY
TEL: +44 (0)20 7359 2244
FAX: +44 (0)20 7359 1616
EMAIL: mail@mqpublications.com
WEBSITE: www.mqpublications.com

Copyright © MQ Publications Limited 2005
Text copyright © Alan Gordon 2005

EDITOR: Karen Ball
DESIGN CONCEPT: Balley Design Associates
DESIGNER: Jo Hill
PHOTOGRAPHY: Mike Prior
ILLUSTRATIONS: Oxford Designers and Illustrators

ISBN: 0-681-27881-1

1 3 5 7 9 0 8 6 4 2

Printed in China

contents

foreword

"We are limited only by what we perceive our horizons to be."

I have written this book to help the ordinary man or woman enjoy the substantial health benefits of increased joint and muscular mobility in a mode of relaxed, safe progress. It is about improving basic flexibility, and does not extend into areas of flexibility training that are very advanced, extensively time-consuming, and highly involved.

New medical evidence is constantly revealing the highly significant link between unexercised, immobile bodies and increasing poor health. As individuals, we are leading busier and fuller lives, and so the need to be healthier and fitter is becoming a necessity rather than a luxury. It is calculated that if we are generally inactive, we will begin to lose our flexibility at around 19–22 years of age. That is a disturbingly early time of life to be relinquishing our full ranges of motion and physical dexterity.

Our early ancestors had very vigorous physical lives, with farming, hunting, and hard manual labor forming part of their daily routine, and so the problems induced by leading a static and sedentary lifestyle simply did not occur. We, however, in our high-tech age of machines and gadgets that do our work for us, cars to drive to and from work, and little leisure time for sport or active hobbies, are in danger of suffering just such problems with our flexibility.

Yet, all you need do to reverse this trend is respect and look after your own body, giving it the exercise it needs. Your body is a truly phenomenal piece of natural engineering: The loading strain capacity of the thigh ligaments and tendons is measured in tons, and despite all the high-tech expertise that surrounds and amazes us these days, the strongest structure known to science is still the human foot! If this wonderful body you were born into is exercised and maintained, it will thrive and respond well to your efforts, giving, in return, a balance and capability that will defy the passing years.

Learning to be more comfortably flexible in order to improve your health requires no tedious feat of learning and memorizing medical and anatomical terminology. Anybody of any age, at anytime and anywhere can do it, and feel significantly better as a result. Once you learn the fundamental lessons and techniques taught within this book, you will automatically have taken out one of the most effective health enhancement policies of your life. And discovering your own flexibility potential is often a revelatory and surprising experience.

Alan Gordon

the principles of flexibility

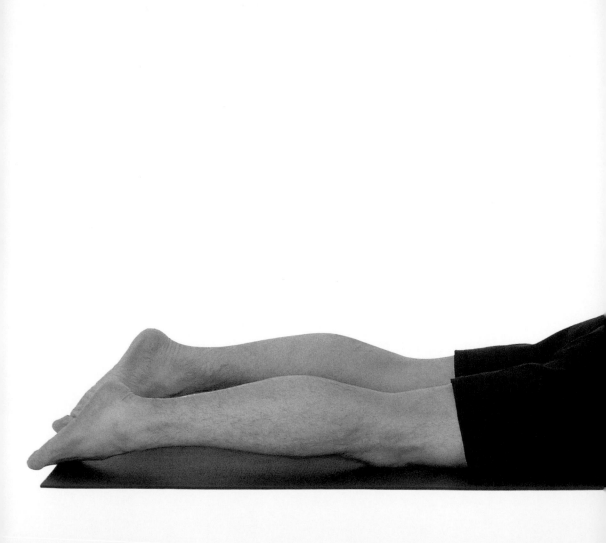

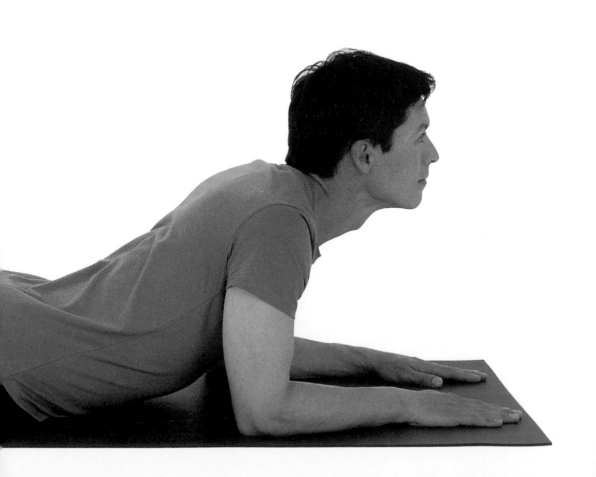

flexibility for you

Whether you are a novice or intermediate trainer, you need a series of foundational flexibility techniques that will give you good basic fitness. Using the information and exercises supplied here, you should be able to develop your training without any hidden cost to your muscles, joints, and ligaments.

As an author, I am unable to see you in the flesh and therefore cannot view any physical idiosyncrasies you may have. I do not know what your motion limitations and restrictions are, and it may well be that your body is totally unsuitable for more advanced stretches. You might, for example, have been born with a slight tilt to your pelvis, or unknowingly have long-established subtle but significant restrictions in your lower/middle spine, both of which conditions would affect how high you could raise your legs.

Despite that lack of knowledge, I can provide you with a range of basic and essential flexibility techniques that will focus your mind and body, providing safe and structured practice. Via these exercises you will slowly discover your own subtle range of motion limitations and joint–muscle restrictions, and you will learn to operate safely within your own parameters. By working through a solid foundational basic flexibility program, you will remain safe while becoming progressively healthier and more invigorated.

Every stretch in this book will work for any sport and for any person: it is as simple as that. The beauty of the selectively safe range of basic flexibility stretches presented here is that they can be developed to a very high degree in their own right, and will make you admirably flexible without any joint, muscle, or ligament problems occurring.

right > **Safe stretching depends upon careful work through gradual stretches. Follow the stretch exercises in this book safely and you will have a good flexibility framework with which to work.**

pacing yourself

We are here to explore basic flexibility through stretch, and it is important to understand that the pace has to be slow and careful. Pushing yourself beyond the biomechanical and physiological safety of your natural level can have significant negative consequences, such as muscle or joint injury.

People often suffer these injuries when they are offered too large a range of flexibility techniques to choose from. With flexibility, as with most things in life, less is more.

Human nature being what it is, the urge to try everything new as soon as possible can lead to small parameters being overlooked.

In short, you may be tempted to push yourself too far, which could result in a potent physiological time bomb that is ready to self-activate at a later stage. A few weeks or months into the future, and a spinal disc twinge or lower back muscle pull could be your reward.

assessing your level

It may be that you are a pretty active person who has already been doing some stretching. But have you been doing it properly, or have you been holding your stretches for far too short a time at the wrong "sensation" point?

Have you, for example, been walking around while stretching your rear upper arms? If you have, you need to take serious stock of your present regime and go back to the effective basic foundations presented in this book, because in the properly safe and long-term subclinically trauma-free sense, I can virtually guarantee that you are still a beginner and should therefore stick to basics.

You may be someone who does what are sometimes referred to as "spontaneous" or "casual" stretches, such as neck stretches made while talking on the telephone, or leg stretches done while reading a newspaper. These are not, however, particularly constructive stretches. All quality flexibility work needs a good degree of concentration to give you a return for your efforts. If you are reading a newspaper or concentrating on a telephone conversation, I guarantee that you

will lose any benefit of the stretch, because of the distractions. If a stretch is worth doing, it is worth doing properly, so allocate sufficient time and concentrate on your basic flexibility training to get the best from it.

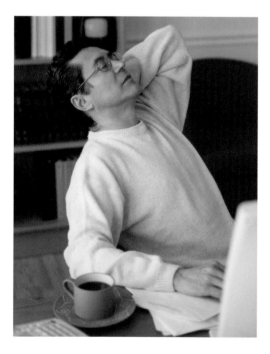

right > **Stretching at your desk is not a good idea. To gain the full benefits of a flexibility program you need to devote concentrated time to your stretch routine, away from day-to-day distractions.**

moving to more advanced training

Much is written about the importance of sport-specific stretches, which are not only crafted around a person's chosen area of training but are also usually engineered to the physiological make-up of that individual.

In other words, "sport specific" in its true sense should also indicate "person specific." While professional sportspeople certainly need a carefully structured program of flexibility training, it is more important for amateurs to concentrate on devising a simple flexibility routine that works well for them and is, most importantly, safe.

It may be that in the future you will choose to move on to more advanced flexibility training, but in order to move on safely to higher levels, you need the sort of good grounding in the basic principles of flexibility that is supplied here. If you do decide to advance, I advise you to find a good personal trainer (whose training and experience both span years) to give you a biomechanical range-of-motion test to ensure safe progression into more advanced stretches. Without that test, it is best to stick to the stretches outlined in this book.

left > **If you intend to develop your flexibility routine further, it is a good idea to source a well-qualified personal trainer.**

establishing your current level of flexibility

We all have to start somewhere and everybody has varying levels of natural flexibility. In order to give yourself a reasonable understanding of where you are at the beginning of your journey to greater ranges of motion and a more supple body, here are three simple procedures to let you know where you stand in the major areas. I'm sure I don't have to remind you that you should not attempt any of these test procedures if you suffer from any relevant injuries or medical conditions, particularly orthopedic spinal problems. If you have any doubts, it is always best to consult your doctor or a suitably qualified fitness professional beforehand.

upper back and chest

Sit on a chair with your back close to a table. Make sure you keep your back comfortably straight and both feet are firmly on the floor. Keeping your pelvis and buttocks as still as possible, turn to the left in an attempt to touch the table behind you with both hands. Repeat this process, turning to the right.

a. If you're not remotely near getting even one hand on the table, you have lots of flexibility work to do on the chest and upper back.

b. If you can get both hands on the table in a 1 o'clock position (or 11 o'clock if turning from the right), you have a respectable level of flexibility.

c. If you can get both hands on the table in a 2 o'clock position (10 o'clock if turning from the right), congratulations, you have good levels of flexibility in the chest and upper back regions.

shoulders and partial chest

Place one elbow behind your head with the hand reaching towards the middle of your back. Pass your other arm past your side also towards the middle of your back and try to interlink the fingers of both hands behind you.

a. If the fingers of each hand don't remotely get near each other, focused flexibility work on the shoulders and chest would be of great benefit to you here.

b. If you're able to touch the fingers of both hands, you have some promising suppleness, but there is still work to do.

c. If you can actually interlink your fingers, you have a good standard of flexibility.

rear upper thighs and lower back

Testing these areas is achieved by simply trying to tie your shoelaces! From a normal standing position, very carefully bend forward from the hips down toward your feet. Keep your knees very slightly bent as you do and make absolutely sure you stop immediately at the first sign of discomfort.

a. If you can't get anywhere near your feet with your hands, then your lower back and rear upper thigh muscles need some serious work.

b. If you can actually tie your shoelaces, well done, you have a respectable level of flexibility—without any difficulty.

c. If you can touch the floor fully with both hands, with your palms down, great stuff. Your flexibility is very good.

flexibility for sport

Whatever sport you play, it is important that you are fully flexible if you are to avoid possible injury. A pre-activity warm-up followed by some stretching is a vital form of preparation, and equally important is a post-activity cool-down and further stretching.

warming-up and cooling-down

It is not nearly good enough to stroll around, windmill your arms a bit, grab your foot and pull it back behind you for a few seconds, then bend forward from the waist—again for just a few seconds—as many soccer players do before a match starts.

In fact, this superficial practice of warm-up stretches before sport events or other physical activities is now coming under fire, particularly when athletes are failing to stretch the larger muscle groups sufficiently.

Emerging evidence reveals that there are greater chances of pulling muscles in large muscle groups if there has been pre-sport activity stretching in these larger groups, particularly the rear upper thighs. Athletes are not always pursuing a thorough warm-up before the event, and are also failing to stretch thoroughly afterward, which all trainers would agree promotes flexibility and injury prevention.

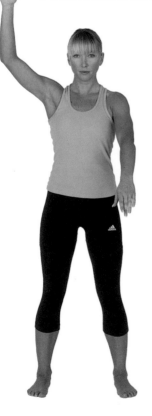

below > **Gentle warm-up stretches should be practised before any sports or vigorous physical activities.**

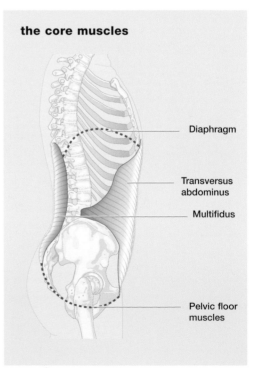

the core muscles

Diaphragm

Transversus abdominus

Multifidus

Pelvic floor muscles

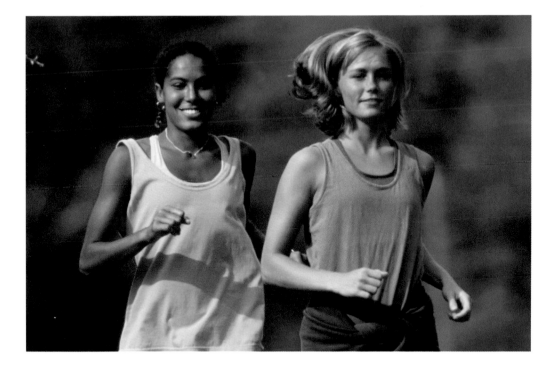

above > **Runners should concentrate on stretching their leg muscles prior to activity.**

Incidents of sprinters falling down in pain, holding their rear upper thigh, just yards from the starting blocks owing to early powerful contractions there seem to substantiate such concerns. If you are an active exerciser or sports participant, and you suffer repeated rear upper thigh or lower leg muscle pulls or muscular problems of this nature on a significantly regular basis, you might care to try out the "no stretch before, only after" approach to training.

order of stretching

With all sports, it is the larger muscle groups that need the most attention, as they provide the greatest "drive." This is why flexibility tutors attend to the legs first (front and rear thigh), then the back (upper and lower), the chest, and finally the arms. Also, within these areas

the stronger muscles are also exercised first, e.g., the front upper arm muscles, then the rear ones.

The emphasis may be changed by the amount of time you spend exercising each muscle group. For example, if you participate in sports that are torso-oriented, such as racket activities, you might want to spend more time on your arms and shoulders, while if you engage in track and distance running, you would put most of your flexibility and stretch efforts into your legs.

It remains a wise decision, however, whether you do this before or after your exertions, to make sure you stretch your "core," which is your lower back and abdominal muscles. This area is the middle link in the chain of three (torso, midsection, and pelvis/legs), and it is involved in literally every single twitch, contraction, or movement you make. In addition, as the connecting "link," it is the most important area in terms of stability during movement.

the main muscle groups

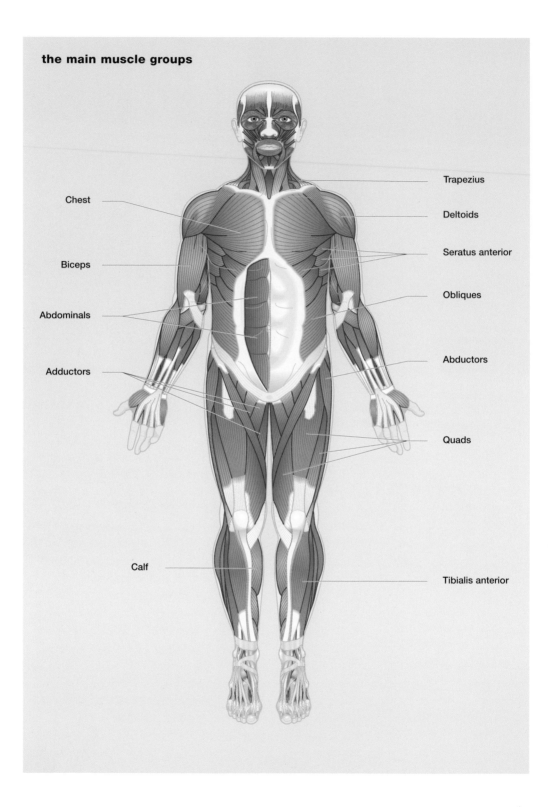

Trapezius

Chest

Deltoids

Seratus anterior

Biceps

Obliques

Abdominals

Adductors

Abductors

Quads

Calf

Tibialis anterior

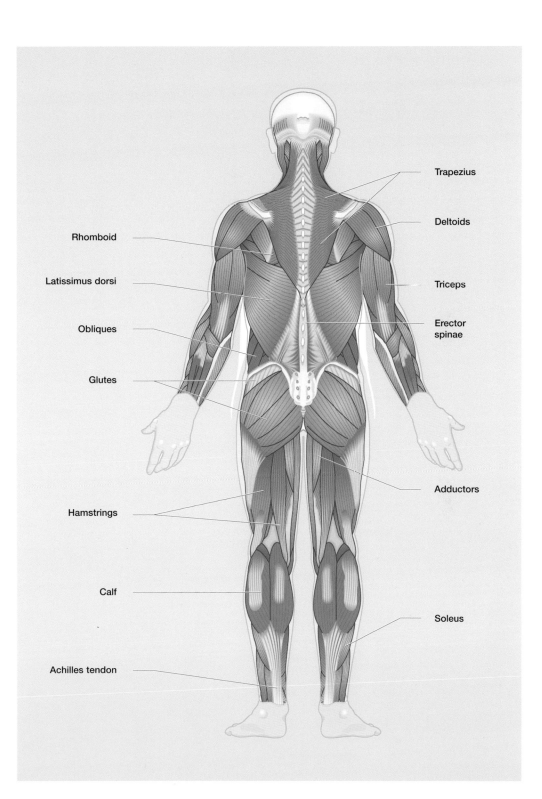

Rhomboid

Latissimus dorsi

Obliques

Glutes

Hamstrings

Calf

Achilles tendon

Trapezius

Deltoids

Triceps

Erector
spinae

Adductors

Soleus

torso versus non-torso sports

When considering sports for basic stretch and flexibility techniques, they break down into two groups: those that use the torso and those that do not.

For example, American football, badminton, basketball, cross-country skiing, hockey, lacrosse, rugby, squash, swimming, tennis, and volleyball are all sports that actively involve the shoulders, arms, and legs, despite the predominance of the legs. Meanwhile, backpacking, cycling, hiking, high jump, orienteering, running, soccer, and triple jump are examples of activities that dominate more strongly with just the legs, since the torso components are not actively contributing to the direct execution of that sport.

The type of training, skills, strength, and stamina that an individual (of whatever size) brings to these different sports is irrelevant. Whether they are a strong 250 lb (113 kg) rugby forward or a lithe and less robust 125 lb

(57 kg) badminton player, a skilful 170 lb (77 kg) soccer player or a highly trained 140 lb (63 kg) long-distance runner, the sports person is still stretching and using the same muscles.

Both the rugby player and the badminton player use their upper body muscles directly as part of what they do, and so will concentrate on shoulder, chest, and arm stretches. Choosing two stretches for each part of the shoulders, chest, and arms and one for each part of the legs, then finishing with their abdominals, is fine. While some people might argue that the differing demands of the sports mean that a rugby player's stretches should be dramatically different from those of a badminton player, there is no clinical evidence for this. The important fact is that

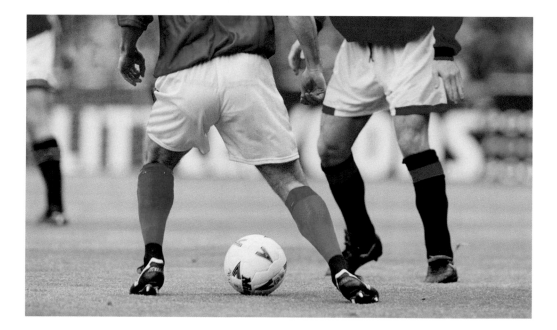

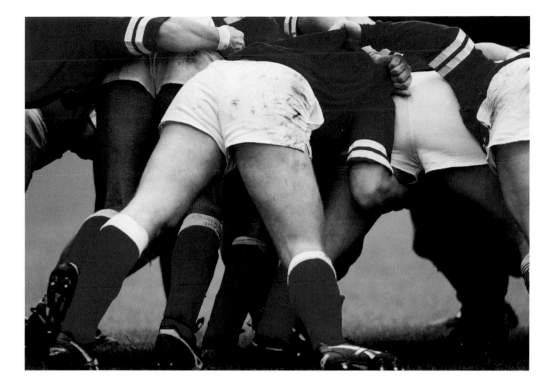

they both use their torsos in their activities, and so both players will benefit from stretches devised for either one of them.

Meanwhile, the soccer player's and runner's upper bodies are very much secondary to what they do, so they should concentrate a little more on the leg and back stretches, with an abdominal finish. They could also put in one arm, shoulder, and upper back stretch if they have time, though this is not a priority. Once again, their stretch exercises are interchangeable.

The bottom line here is that basic flexibility is all about stretching muscles—how powerful they are, how tall or short you are, and how weak or strong you are is irrelevant. What the muscles are used for does not matter at all. You are trying to make yourself more flexible and injury-free, working within the controls of your body and personal ranges of motion, to lengthen your muscles and ease your joints.

left and above > **Rugby and soccer concentrate on different parts of the body: rugby actively involves the upper body, whereas soccer players' lower bodies are utilized much more than their upper bodies.**

Once you know which groups of muscles to concentrate on, you will be able to devise your own stretch routine and choose your own mixture of stretches from the ones provided in this book.

In all stretch regimes, progression is achieved more readily by extending time spent at your "annoying ache" (or "AA") point. This is a term I use for the point in a stretch where you can feel the effect on your body. It is more than a mild pull but not so extreme as to be painful. The sensation of the ache marks the productive stage of the stretch, and you should aim to hold a stretch for 60–90 seconds in this position.

how to arrange your flexibility routine

Any torso muscle that is directly contracted against any load beyond limb weight alone needs more stretching, as the load borne (whatever form it takes) throughout the activity will tighten and exert those muscles far more.

Examples of this are rugby players clutching and dragging their opponents down to the ground, basketball players using their arms and shoulders to move and throw the weight of the basketball around at speed, and hockey players wielding their sticks to move and forcefully strike the hockey ball along the ground. All these are examples of the muscular contractions required being much greater and more demanding than the contractions required to move and maneuver just the limb weight around, as in the case of soccer players, distance runners, or orienteers.

If you engage in activities that exercise the upper body, the greater range of muscles used means that you will need to do more stretching. Once you have performed your warm-up, the stretches will occupy no more than five to eight minutes. (There is an inherent danger with stretches, which are static,

below > **Tennis players use their muscles to bear the load of a racquet and hit the tennis ball at speed. This type of exercise can exert muscles far more than sports that only require the person to move themselves around.**

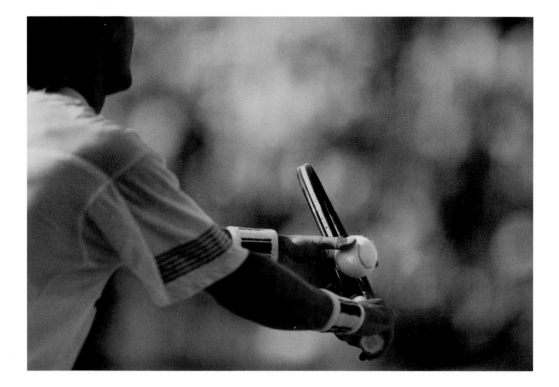

because standing and lying still for too long can lead to cooling-down and a loss of the preparatory effect of the warm-up.) However, if you are a devotee of the "only stretch afterward" philosophy, you will have no cool-down considerations to bear in mind. Nevertheless, please remember that you need to stretch your abdominals and your lower back, whatever your sport or activity, and this is regardless of whether you stretch before and after exercising, or only after it.

The aim of this book is to lead your body to a state of good basic flexibility using a selective and fairly moderate number of stretches. The postures, alignments, and ranges are specifically chosen because of their noncompressive nature on any of the joints (particularly the spinal column). They involve reasonable ranges of motion, even for the absolute novice, and allow you, if you wish, to develop the scope of the stretches to a much higher level of flexibility, without in any way losing the safety they provided on the day you first attempted them.

There are a great many more advanced flexibility techniques available, and there is no reason, once you have developed your flexibility beyond the scope of this book, why you should not progress to these. Mastering the postures and techniques in this book first means that you will have established an excellent and competent level of basic flexibility. From this basis, you can go forward in the certain knowledge that your body is completely ready to face more demanding criteria, and that you are physically capable of taking that next step in flexibility with confidence and experience.

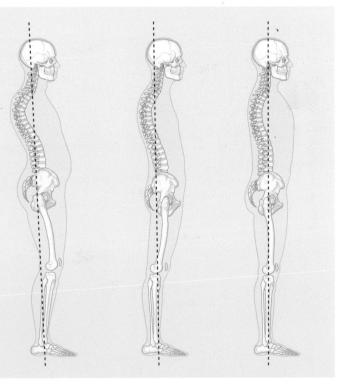

posture

Good spinal posture is important in rest and in play. Working to improve your day-to-day posture will help you achieve a good range of motion in the sport you choose to play. The middle diagram opposite shows good, relaxed standing posture, with poor posture on the left and an overly rigid spine posture on the far right.

the benefits of stretching

So you are stretching, it feels good, and that's terrific. Then someone turns to you and says, "Yes, but what's happening and why do you feel good?" Replying that stretching relaxes your mind and body is certainly an adequate answer, but there are also definite clinical benefits to your physique taking place, which are explained below.

protecting against injuries

Stretching is a first-class defense system against injuries, because the greater your ranges of motion and the more flexible your muscular system is, the less likely you are to suffer sprains or pulls when muscles are unexpectedly twisted or made to move quickly in any direction. It is a plain fact of physiology that an unstretched muscle, however strong, is significantly less able to withstand stress than a muscle that is flexible and supple. Not only that, but another law of physiology states that "the more you stretch a muscle, the more powerfully it contracts." This means that if a muscle is flexible and is able to stretch comfortably to a greater degree, when that muscle returns back from the stretch to its resting state, it is able to contract even more powerfully, therefore resulting in greater strength and capability.

improving circulation

Stretching improves your circulation. When anything is tight and contracted, the resulting pressure is obviously greater, and the human circulatory system is no exception. Tight, inflexible muscles constrict blood vessels and impair efficient circulation, not to mention contributing to raised blood pressure. By making the muscle more flexible, you increase the suppleness of the fibers, and so the load on the circulation is significantly reduced, which is good for your heart, skin, muscles, and general health.

warming-up and cooling-down

Stretching makes all activity easier, as the process automatically signals a readiness for activity, if you are about to undertake any exercise. However, this does not mean that if you are stretching simply to relax, you create an unwanted, heightened anticipation that tenses you up. The fact is that the stretch process has a dual effect: It can both prepare you for action and calm you down, which is another pretty remarkable characteristic of the flexibility process.

becoming aware

Stretching helps you develop an awareness of your body. As your stretch techniques and abilities develop, the "awareness" factor occurs. The best way to describe this is to imagine that, when you begin, you say to yourself, "I'm going to stretch my rear upper thigh" (hamstrings) and you try to focus on that area alone. As a beginner, you will get a reasonable feel of isolating that area to do the job. However, in a relatively short period of time, smoothly and almost without thinking about it, your awareness begins to escalate. The regular habit of flexibility training allows you to become much more aware of the limits and abilities of your body, which parts of your body work best, and how they are improving. For possibly the first time in your life, you are paying focused attention to the body you inhabit. You will find that you can focus on any area of your body with a precision and

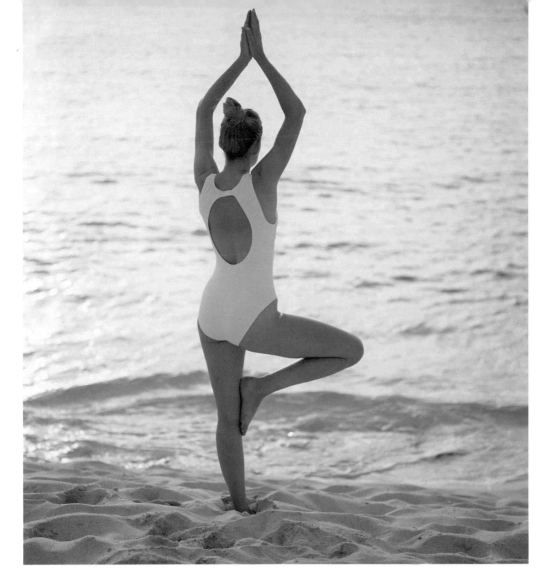

exactness that will surprise you. Your body awareness has arrived…and is here to stay.

decreasing tension

Stretching decreases both physiological and psychological tension. The link between the body and mind is well established, and it is recognized that the state of mind and levels of focus in any sport affect the physical results. The opposite is also true: the body can influence the mind. Stretching for greater flexibility releases tension, and after a really bad, stressful day at work, a stretch routine in which your body flows into natural relaxation

above > **Sports therapists have long recognized the strong link between mental and physical health. A good stretch routine can help you mentally and emotionally relax.**

rhythms is precisely what the doctor ordered. Performed regularly, stretching can calm the system and destress very tense and busy people to a positive, remedial degree that can improve their overall health. Stretching areas such as the very large back and neck muscle (trapezius), which inserts at the base of the skull, can often rid you of obvious signs of stress such as a headache.

when to stretch

You can increase your flexibility at any hour of the day, but you do need to be aware of how the time of day affects your movement. Your ranges of motion and muscular release abilities vary at two points in the day—first, early morning and second, late morning/mid-afternoon onward—and for this reason, care must be taken not to apply your late afternoon range of motion limitations to an early morning stretch session.

air pressure

Air pressure measures 15 lb per sq. in. (2.7 kg per sq. cm.), and this weight is bearing down upon you all the time. It is not something you are ever aware of as you go about your daily routine, but it equates to quite a hefty weight to carry around. Knowing about air pressure helps you understand why when you get a bad back of some description, it aches a lot even when you are not doing anything. Except you are—you are carrying the weight of all that air around. Air pressure is also an important factor regarding when you exercise.

early morning

When you wake up in the morning, after a normal and restful night's sleep, a number of conditions are in play:

● Your muscular system, joints, and ligaments are very relaxed.

● You are, on average, ⅛ in. (3–4 mm) taller for the first five to ten minutes of walking around. This is due to the opening out of the spinal column's intervertebral discs when you were lying down all night. These discs have been allowed to expand and open up to their full unpressured size during the night, through not having to contend with their daytime job of supporting your posture in an upright position.

● Your entire system, for the first 20 minutes or so of moving around in the morning, is adjusting to air pressure on the spinal column, which in turn conveys pressure to your knee joints and feet.

● Your muscles are adjusting to all your movement rhythms, which have been almost static all night. There will therefore be certain movement restrictions, and the need to stretch out like a cat when it wakes up after a nap is commonly mimicked by us in the classic yawn and splayed-arms-above-the-head posture.

This is a time when you need to take care if you decide to enjoy an early stretch session to loosen up for the coming day. Always bear in mind that your muscular stretch limits where those stretches are comfortably achieved will be less than during the late morning or afternoon/evening.

late morning onward

By late morning, you will probably have moved around considerably and your body will have mobilized itself into the daily schedule. It will nearly always be capable of greater stretch ranges of motion from this time onward, however small they might be, even if you are a regular flexibility devotee.

stretching after exercise

Flexibility through stretching is also a great ally in the battle against muscular soreness after activity. It is instrumental in easing stiffness in the muscles after any prolonged exercise.

From roller-painting the ceiling to running a marathon, it always helps and brings relief. Later, I will discuss in greater depth how and why it does this, and detail a range of activities in which to apply your new skills.

air pressure on the spine

The spinal column is always carrying weight in the form of air pressure. This compresses the space between the intervertebral discs.

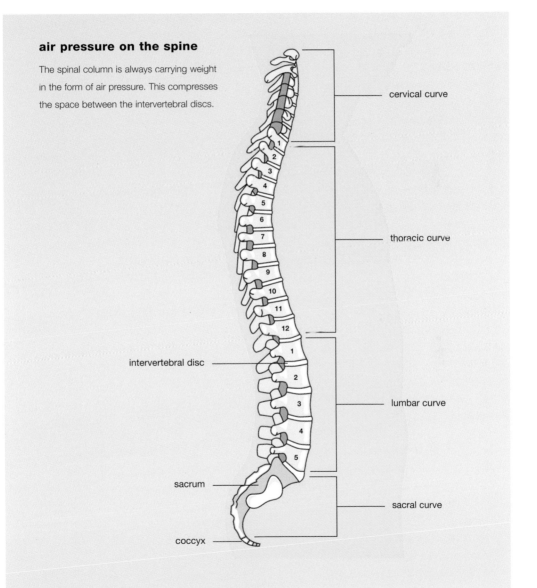

cervical curve

thoracic curve

intervertebral disc

lumbar curve

sacrum

sacral curve

coccyx

flexibility technique

Stretching to increase your flexibility is a very easy technique to learn, but there is a right and a wrong way to do it. The right way is to maintain a sustained and relaxed stretch, with your mind focused on the muscle(s) you are trying to stretch. The wrong way is to bounce up and down (known as "ballistic" stretching), when it is all too easy to bounce to a point where, regardless of how short a time you are there, you are in pain.

feeling the AA point

When you begin, stretch gently until you feel a mild sensation of resistance and tension in the target muscle, then hold. Remember that tension point and call it the "annoying ache" point (AA). The AA will gradually move away from you as the muscle stretches, and it is perfectly acceptable to pursue it gently. When you hold the AA, the feeling of tension should ease off; and when you are sure that it has eased, then—and only then—you can ease further in the tiniest fractions of movement until you reach your AA again. You must be in absolute control throughout this process.

breathing properly

Throughout your flexibility stretching techniques, your breathing should be relaxed, rhythmic, and controlled. Never hold your breath while stretching. If your breathing is impaired by your stretch position, then you are not relaxed and you need to reposition yourself so you can breathe properly. If you are involved in a stretch that requires you to bend forward, exhale as you lower yourself and breathe slowly as you hold that stretch.

timing yourself

To get the best results from your flexibility training, you need to be aware of time and the number of seconds that are involved in giving you a properly efficient result in your endeavors. Often you are advised just to count

slowly, estimating the seconds, but to be absolutely certain that you are maximizing your time fully, use a watch or a clock with a second hand. Guessing is all very well, but it is much more fruitful and satisfying when you can plainly see that you spent the right amount of time in each stretch, rather than be left wondering later if you miscounted at some point. Timing is very important indeed.

the myotatic and inverse myotatic reflexes

The real benefit of a stretch begins only after 15 seconds of stretching at the AA. This is the starting point of quality returns on your investment, so 30 seconds of stretch delivers 15 seconds of "value for money."

There are two reflexes involved in the stretching process: the myotatic reflex and the inverse myotatic reflex:

● The *myotatic* reflex allows a muscle to stretch out unhindered. It is fairly obvious, however, that a muscle being allowed to stretch out completely unhindered is not safe, since at some point this would result in a muscle tear as it reached its maximum length and kept on going into the damage zone.

● The inverse *myotatic* reflex puts a brake on the momentum of the myotatic, and stops the stretch process safely at a point before any damage is incurred.

When you stretch to the AA, this is where the myotatic has reached its furthest safety point, and the inverse myotatic stops it moving further for the sake of damage limitation and establishing acceptable levels of muscle and ligament lengthening. Beyond the point where the inverse myotatic has brought matters to a halt (at what you feel is the AA) is a damage zone, and when a stretch is forced past this line of mild tension, it is painful.

As the flexibility of the muscle increases, the inverse myotatic allows the myotatic a little more freedom, but only when it is safe to do so. This is what happens during your stretch when you are pursuing your AA as it recedes a fraction further away from you, until you reach the maximum levels of your flexibility threshold at that stage of your development.

ballistic stretching

"Ballistic," or bounce, stretching is where you use momentum to help the myotatic literally bounce the muscle repeatedly past the safety line established by the inverse myotatic. The damage done (known as subclinical micro-trauma) is often not evident at first, as it is a very subtle ongoing process. Small muscle fibers are torn each time the ballistic approach is used, and because the damage is so subtle, it goes unheeded in the immediate sense.

However, this form of damage gradually accumulates and develops from subclinical micro-trauma to clinical trauma, which is damage that you are very much aware of, and which causes considerable pain. The change occurs when the unseen damage has built up and up until one day the point is reached where that last step is taken, and suddenly

you have an injury that will cause you considerable discomfort, certainly curtail your activities, and may well require the attentions of a physiotherapist.

Ballistic stretching is a conscious and determined course of action that actually undermines your own defense system. Practicing it therefore means that you are knowingly doing something that is unsafe and that can cause you injury if you persist with it. The message is quite simple: don't do it.

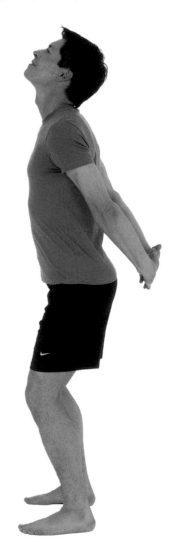

right > **Your own body will tell you the extent to which you should take a stretch: the AA point, or "annoying ache" will let you know not to take a stretch further.**

healthy eating and flexibility

All exercise should be supplemented by a healthy diet, but this can be particularly true for flexibility. Light, regular meals are the best option for anyone who stretches regularly, and you should not eat for two hours before any extended program of stretching.

Feeding the body can improve flexibility. It is well established that the fatty acids found in oily fish, such as salmon, help joint flexibility. Healthy eating keeps you trim, which allows you to move into positions more easily, and a healthy body means a healthy mind, so good eating habits allow the stress-relieving benefits of flexibility training to have even more impact. It goes without saying that a good attitude toward food will help your flexibility training, but it is not always easy to introduce new eating habits into your lifestyle.

When you are cooking at home, it is a great deal easier to stick to a healthy diet. Buy a good lowfat cookbook, make sure your kitchen is stocked with healthy food, and banish all convenience foods from your cupboards. Restrict snacking to fruit and vegetables. What is much harder is sticking to the straight and narrow when you are eating in a restaurant, where temptation is all around you. Below I have outlined some guidelines that should make that food selection process easier, without depriving yourself completely.

simple guide to eating out more healthily

Imagine your meal as being divided into three equal parts:
- About one-third of the meal should be some form of lean protein (fish, chicken, tofu, etc.)
- Up to one-third of the meal should come from complex carbohydrates (brown rice, sweet potato, beans, etc.)
- At least one-third of the meal should consist of fibrous vegetables (salad, broccoli, etc.)

Now order accordingly.

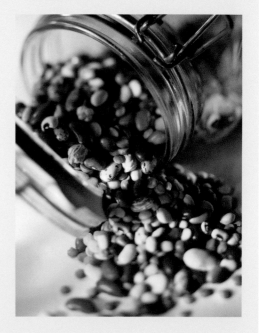

Before the meal:
- Ask for water immediately, and drink it.
- If you are drinking alcohol, choose wine, and alternate with water.
- Skip the bread, tortillas, and other "free" nibbles that are brought to the table before the meal.
- If you cannot resist the bread, eat it without butter. If you must have something with your bread, ask for extra-virgin olive oil to dip it into.

Appetizers:
- Ask for salad dressings on the side. Then, taste the salad without the dressing. Acceptably good? Then skip the dressing. If not, try dipping your fork in the dressing first, then picking up a mouthful of food with your "dipped" utensil.
- Avoid fried anything.
- Choose vegetable, bean, or tomato-based soups.
- Ask for raw vegetable platters with non-creamy dips—these are becoming more widely available on request in restaurants.
- Steamed seafood or prawn salads are another good option.

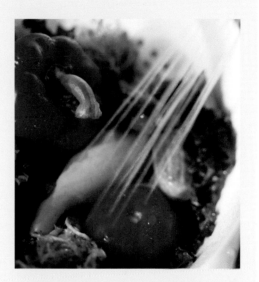

Main courses:
- Avoid white sauces, or anything made with cream.
- Choose broiled or baked meats in no sauce (or a light sauce).
- Ask if your meal can be prepared without butter.
- If you order chicken, ask for skinless breast, if possible.
- When eating Italian, consider passing on pasta for a fish or chicken dish.
- If you order pasta as a main course, choose one with chicken or fish, or ask if it can be added.

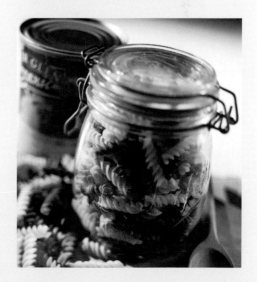

Side dishes:

- Always choose a vegetable side dish with your meal.
- Choose brown rice instead of potatoes.
- If you do choose potatoes, mashed or boiled are best. Always eat them without butter, cheese, or sour cream—if you must add a dressing to a baked potato, make it cottage cheese.
- Order vegetables steamed or raw.
- Pass on potato salad and pasta salad as side dishes. Ask for fruit, salad, or steamed vegetables instead.
- Plain noodles, rice pilaf, or mushrooms cooked in wine are also healthy options.

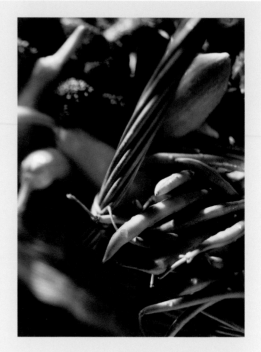

Desserts:

- Make dessert an occasional treat rather than the natural end to every meal.
- If you have dessert, the best choice is fresh fruit—but without cream.
- Other good choices for dessert include fruit ices, sorbets, and frozen yogurts.
- Try splitting a dessert with a friend.
- Beware of milky coffee drinks. They can be full of fat and calories. Try flavored coffees or drinks made with skim milk rather than cream.

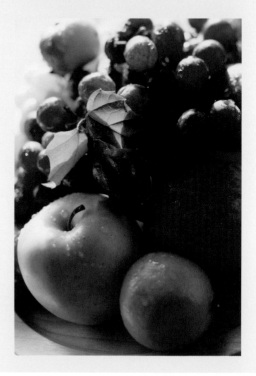

keep a food diary

The best way to begin a healthy eating program is by keeping a record of everything you eat in one week. This puts you in control of your own eating habits and makes you more conscious of exactly what you eat and why. It is a good idea to add notes to your diary recording where and when you eat your meals and what mood you are in each day— perhaps you will discover that you only snack on chocolate and crisps when you are bored or depressed or that you only eat junk food when you are out with friends.

days	breakfast	lunch	dinner	snacks	notes
monday					
tuesday					
wednesday					
thursday					
friday					
saturday					
sunday					

stress management and flexibility

One of the reasons for starting a stretch routine is to make yourself less stressed and realize your body's full relaxation potential. However, you first need to address the very important issue of your start condition in order to see how you can make stretch and flexibility work for you.

First of all, you must ask yourself two questions: how stressed are you now and how will basic flexibility help you feel better? Your degree of progress can often depend on how tense you are at the start of your flexibility program. The less anxious you are, the quicker you will feel the benefits of your constructive flexibility routine, and the sooner concerns such as tension headaches, short temper, and fatigue are improved.

understanding stress

Stress is the wear and tear our bodies experience as we adjust to our continually changing environment. It has physical and emotional effects on us and can create both positive and negative feelings.

positive stress

As a positive influence, stress can help compel us to action and it can also result in a new vitality, which often creates an exciting and more invigorated outlook on life. Positive stress, known as "eucontistress," or "eu-stress" adds anticipation and excitement to our lives, and we all actually thrive under a certain amount of this positive stress. Deadlines, competitions, confrontations, and sometimes even our lesser frustrations all add greater depth and diversity to our lives.

negative stress

As a negative influence, stress can result in feelings of distrust, rejection, anger, and depression, which in turn can lead to health problems such as headaches, upset stomachs, rashes, insomnia, ulcers, high blood pressure, heart disease, and stroke. Excessive negative stress may leave us feeling physically contracted, with a pronounced feeling of being tied up in knots. This is where flexibility and stretch routines can be of enormous assistance.

getting the balance right

Your goal should not be to eliminate stress completely (insufficient eu-stress can act like a depressant and may often leave you feeling bored, dejected, or apathetic). Instead, you need to learn how to manage stress and how to use it in a postive way to help you. What you need to do is find the optimal level of stress: one that will individually motivate you but not be overwhelming.

the clinical realities of stress

Significant negative stress levels can have dramatic biochemical effects on your body. Stress hormones are released, occurring in direct proportion to the level of stress present. The hormones are immune-suppressive and lower the number of your defense cells, so making you more susceptible to infection and illness. Indeed, it has been discovered that vast numbers of illnesses are related to unrelieved stress. The hormones also compromise the body's fuel-processing effects within you, which then renders your entire system prematurely fatigued and abnormally low in available energy levels.

Stress affects your short- and long-term memory, your attention span, and your physical coordination. There is also new evidence that strongly suggests that stress may affect the protective "insulation" that covers all the nerve fibers in your body (called the myelin sheath). It may also create biochemical conditions within you that are favorable for the development of numerous different cancers.

finding your optimal stress level

There is no single level of stress that is optimal for everyone. What is very distressing to one person may be stimulating to another, and even when a number of people agree that a particular event causes stress, they are still likely to differ in their physiological and psychological responses to it. For example, if you love to arbitrate disputes and move from job to job, you would be irritatingly stressed in an occupation that was stable and routine, and vice versa. In addition, your personal stress requirements and the amounts you can tolerate before you actually become distressed change with age.

If you are experiencing definite stress symptoms, then you have gone beyond your optimal stress level and you need to reduce the stress in your life and/or improve your ability to manage it.

below > **Stress can often make itself felt in shoulder and neck muscles that tighten up uncomfortably.**

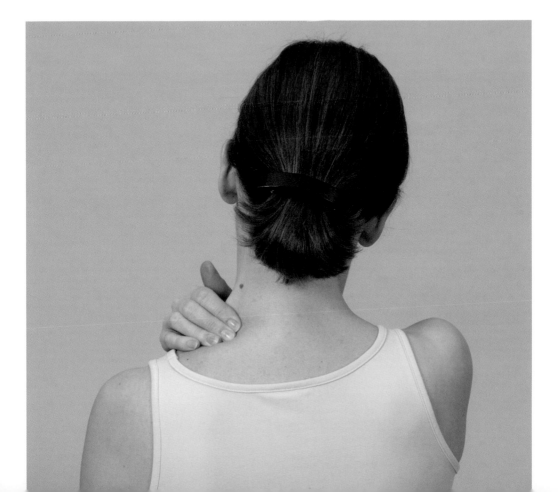

managing stress more effectively

Just identifying unrelieved stress and being aware of its effect on our lives is not sufficient for reducing its harmful effects. Just as there are many sources of stress, so there are many possibilities for its management, such as stretch or meditation. However, they all require effort toward change, namely changing the source of the stress and/or changing your reaction to it. There are six crucial steps to take to achieve this change.

1. Become aware of your stress sources and your emotional and physical reactions to them.

● Address your distress: Do not ever ignore it, and do not gloss over any of your problems.

● Determine which events distress and upset you. What are you telling yourself about the meaning and magnitude of these events?

● Determine how your body responds to the stress. Do you become nervous or physically upset? Do you suffer from headaches, muscular tension, irritability, or "cannot be bothered, too tired" syndrome? Do you become short-tempered or depressed?

2. Recognize what you can change.

● Can you change your stress sources by avoiding or eliminating them completely?

● Can you reduce their intensity by managing them over a longer period of time, instead of on a daily or weekly basis?

● Can you shorten your exposure to stress by taking a break, or physically leaving the premises where you work (if you have discovered it to be part of the problem)?

● Can you devote the time and energy necessary to make a change?

3. Reduce the intensity of your emotional reactions to stress.

● The stress reaction is triggered by your perception of physical and/or emotional danger. Are you viewing your stress in exaggerated terms and turning a normally difficult situation into a full-blown disaster?

● Are you attempting the impossible, i.e., to please everyone?

● Are you overreacting and viewing too many things as absolutely critical and urgent?

● Do you feel you must always come out on top in every situation?

● As much as you can, try to work at adopting more moderate views. Try to see the stress as something you can cope with, instead of something that overpowers you. Also, try hard to moderate what you know to be your excess emotions. Put the situation in perspective rather than dwelling on the negative aspects of the situations in your life.

4. Learn to moderate your physical reactions to stress.

● Slow and controlled deep breathing will bring your heart rate and respiration back to normal, and you will easily be able to develop this in flow with your stretch and flexibility. The flexibility techniques outlined in this book will reduce muscle tension and encourage a calm, restful state.

● If you feel that prescription medicines are absolutely necessary, use them only in the very short term to moderate any dramatic physical reactions. However, they alone are certainly not the answer. Learning to moderate these reactions yourself is undoubtedly the best long-term solution.

5. Look after yourself.

● Relax, shut your eyes, and work on "getting away from it all" by doing a gentle, quiet stretch routine.

● As much as you possibly can, ensure your food intake is well balanced and nutritious.

● Strive to maintain the weight at which you feel your most confident, as your self-esteem is vital.

● Mix leisure with work, taking breaks and getting away whenever it is possible.

● Get enough sleep, and be consistent with your sleep schedule as much as possible.

● Avoid alcohol, and caffeine if you can. If not, try to decrease your intake significantly.

6. Maintain your emotional reserves.

● Pursue realistic goals that are meaningful to you, rather than ones other people impose on you. Always expect some frustrations, failures, and sorrows, as they are unavoidable.

above > **Learning simple meditation techniques is a good way of managing stress.**

● Understand, too, that in its more dramatic stages of development, negative stress most certainly ruins lives and weakens the immune system along with your ability to ward off illnesses and disease. It is therefore very much in the interests of your long-term health and well-being to take charge of any negative stress present in your life. In this way you will strengthen your body's resilience and lay the foundations for a more contented future.

warming-up

The warming-up process for a stretch session to improve flexibility differs from the warm-up for sport or for an activity such as digging the garden. It should match the spirit of the stretch session, which is one of relaxation and getting there by gentle, unhurried means.

The following three activities are all you need to do in order to prepare your body for a stretch session. Almost no one needs instructions for a stretch session warm-up, since it is as simple and uncomplicated as walking around. The all-important word you should always have in your head when warming-up is "gently."

the windmill stretch

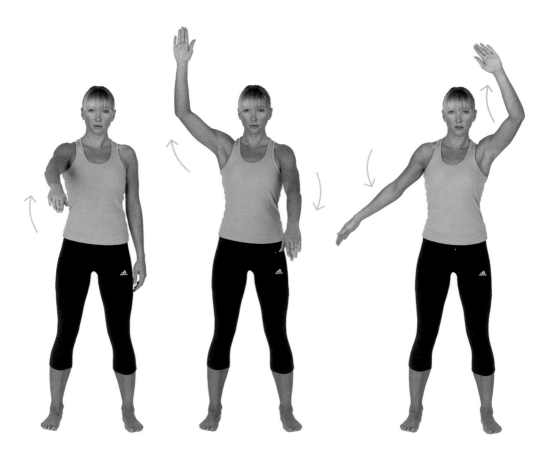

Gently windmill your arms on either side of your torso.

shoulder shrug

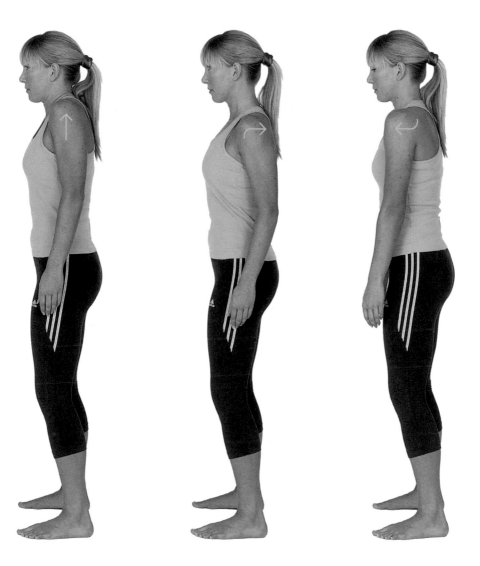

Shrug your shoulders.
Comfortably bend and stretch
gently, up and down, back
and forth.

Now slowly move your arms outward and back
behind you, until you feel the stretch in your chest,
front upper arms, and forearms.

straight leg against wall stretch

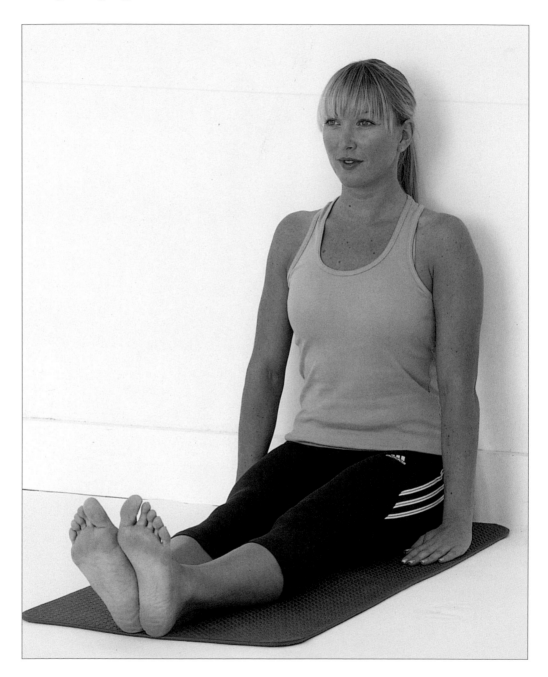

Sit on the floor and gently bend and straighten your legs out
along the carpet.

the physiology of the warm-up process explained

Unless the weather is very humid or extremely hot, you should not break into a sweat. If you do, then you have actually slightly overheated in terms of stretch receptiveness, and this has affected your resting metabolic rate.

To be at its most efficient, blood should remain in the center of a muscle—an area known as the "belly" of the muscle. However, if you exert yourself to a point where you start to sweat, it means that you are dissipating the accumulated heat that you have created and your body is now trying to maintain your bodily core temperature at the right level through perspiration. The harder you exert, the more you sweat, as the more heat there is to divert away from your "core" to sustain the desirable temperature there.

This reaction of the body is all part of the complex survival process known as thermoregulation, which is used by the body to keep the body at a certain temperature despite varying environmental temperatures. Although this gentle warm-up is not, of course, in the least bit dangerous, and therefore does not merit the activation of a survival process, the thermoregulatory system begins its defense actions at even the faintest sign of any irregularity.

Along with this heat evacuation comes the role of the circulatory system. The more you work, the redder you get as the blood is forced to the surface of your body to help evacuate the unwanted heat via the surface of your skin. So, your flushed state means that your blood is not in the bellies of your muscles, where it should be; instead, it's being pushed away from them to cool you down.

Stopping yourself from activating your thermoregulatory system is actually very simple. Nobody really knows your body like you do. Therefore, you will know instinctively just how much gentle movement it takes, allowing for hot, cold, or humid conditions, to make you break into a sweat. Gauge your gentle pre-stretch warm-up to coincide with the temperature around you, and just get pleasantly warm, nothing more.

This will go a long way in helping you start your stretch session more efficiently; and, since you won't have to contend with a dripping face and uncomfortable sticky back, you will be a lot more comfortable, too.

arm and shoulder stretches

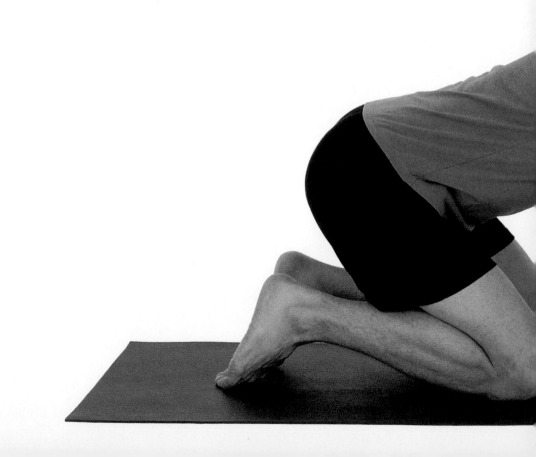

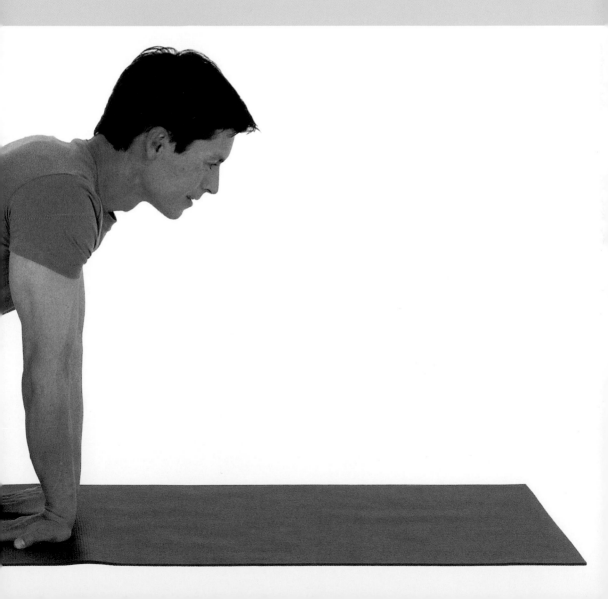

the diver

benefits: This stretch was originally devised to stretch the chest, but with small adjustments it is also an excellent stretch for the biceps and forearms. Its name comes from the fact that the final posture resembles a diver's stance on a high board.

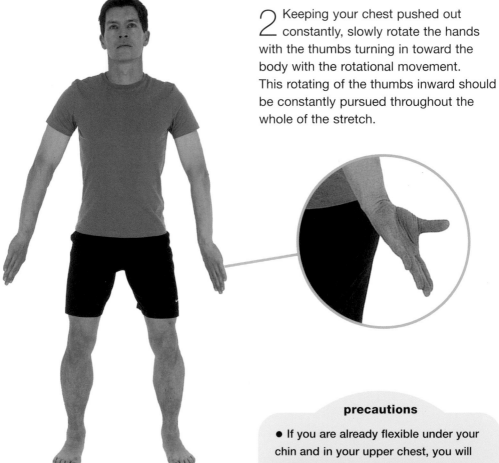

2 Keeping your chest pushed out constantly, slowly rotate the hands with the thumbs turning in toward the body with the rotational movement. This rotating of the thumbs inward should be constantly pursued throughout the whole of the stretch.

1 Stand with your chest thrust out gently and arms straight down by your sides. Make a chopping shape with your hands and extend the thumbs out clear of your fingers.

precautions

● If you are already flexible under your chin and in your upper chest, you will be able to tilt your head back a considerable way, and could be in danger of compressing the back of your neck too much in the process. For this reason, you should always retain an awareness of the back of your neck.

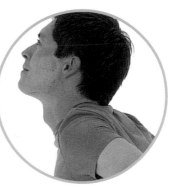

● Keep a sharp eye on the sensations in your front shoulders when you perform this stretch. Women, in particular, are susceptible to subtle damage here. An acute pressurized sensation is something to be avoided here, as a part of your shoulder structure called the "rotator cuff" can be compromised if you don't get to your AA point gently and carefully.

3 Once you have reached this point, gently tilt your head back, looking up and directly back until you feel another stretch at the front of your neck and under your chin.

4 Make minor adjustments to the positioning of your arms, the height at which you take them back behind you or out from your body, and also the degree to which you push your chest out. In this way you will discover that you can shift the focus of the stretch to where you feel you need it most in your flexibility routine. Maintain the AA at your chosen focus point for a minimum of 30 seconds.

forearm stretch

benefits: This is an excellent inner forearm stretch, but one that is often neglected. This lack of attendance can subtly affect the efficiency of the hand grip in racket sports. This is because the contractile abilities of the bicep during the initial stages of an activity have been compromised.

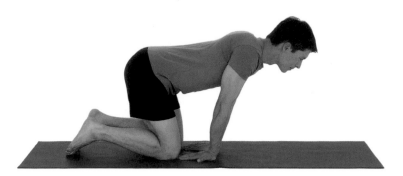

1 Kneel on all fours, supporting yourself on your hands and knees. Rotate your wrists so your thumbs point to the outside and your fingers point back toward your knees.

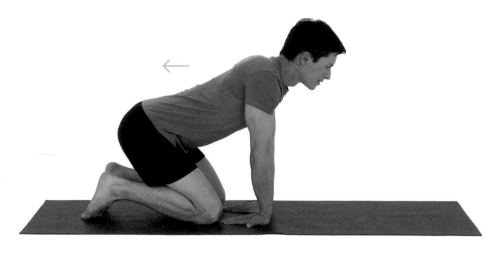

2 Now, very gently and gradually lean back, ensuring you keep your palms flat on the floor as you do so. Lean back only as far as your forearms will allow you to, without sacrificing the total touch of your palms on the floor.

3 Hold at the AA in the inner forearms for a minimum of 30 seconds.

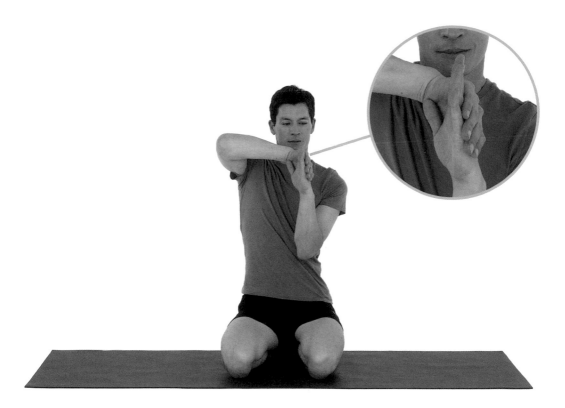

4 In order to release any accumulated tension in the outside
of your wrists, once you have finished this stretch, grip your
left hand with your right and gently push it down and in toward
the wrist. Exert only gentle pressure with your right hand until
you feel the stretch on the outside of your left wrist. Hold this for
30 seconds and repeat with your left hand gripping the right.

precautions

● The angle at the wrists that is required to enact this stretch to
its maximum potential risks overly compressing the wrists on the
outside of the forearms, which can cause problems. For this
reason, you should take great care when moving to the AA.

standing lat stretch

benefits: This very effective stretch is used commonly by bodybuilders to create a more pronounced shape in the latissimus dorsi (lats for short).

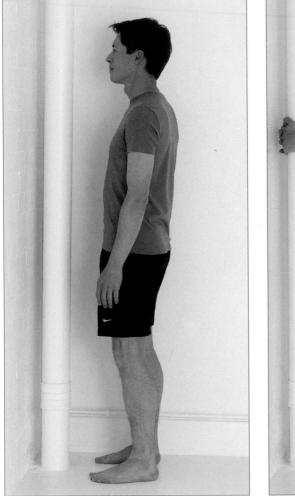
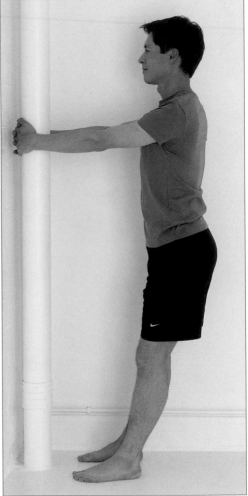

1 Stand with your fingers interlaced around the back of a banister or post—or anything else that you can either comfortably grip or interlace your fingers around for supporting your partial body weight while you lean back—or grip it with your hands. (Interlacing your fingers is usually a more efficient support anchor from which to lean back, but gripping is fine if that is what you prefer.)

● The latissimus dorsi are the muscles of the back that create a V shape (usually far more pronounced in men than in women). These are often very highly developed in bodybuilders.
● The classic early morning standing stretch that so many of us perform when we get up is an unconscious attempt to stretch this particular group of muscles, and the standing lat stretch given here is basically a far more efficient way of getting that early morning "loosening" experience.

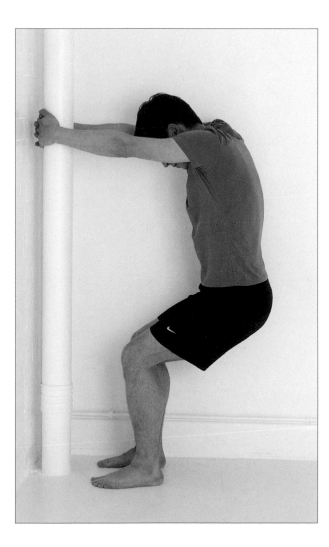

2 Bend at the knees and thrust your bottom out gently behind you. Let your body relax back with your arms perfectly straight, but round your shoulders forward toward the post as you do so. This stretch can be altered to vary its intensity, but your bottom must always be thrust out gently behind you, whatever position you decide to adopt, because it protects your lower back from stress during this flexibility technique.

rear shoulder stretch

benefits: A more flexible and mobile rear shoulder can prevent rhomboid spasms. These spasms, close to the rear shoulder, are often what cause us to wake up with a start and a sharp point of discomfort in the rear shoulder/upper back. Stretching this area will discourage such spasms.

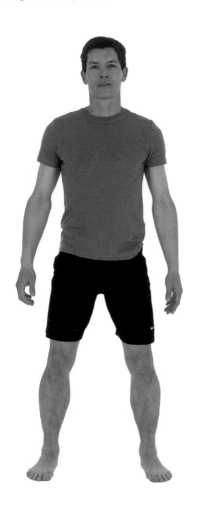

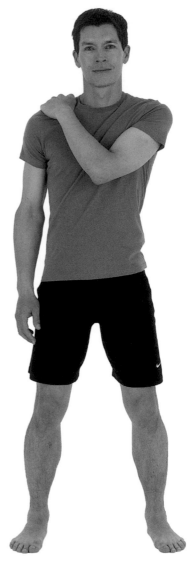

1 Stand with your feet hip-width apart and your arms hanging loosely by your sides.

2 Lift your left arm horizontally across your chest and toward your right shoulder.

3 Clasp your left elbow with your right hand, allowing your left arm to hang completely limp. The relaxed left arm should literally be a dead weight for the supporting and pulling right arm, and you should experience a really pronounced sense of the left shoulder blade lifting off the back.

4 Hold the AA for a minimum of 30 seconds, then repeat with the left arm clasping the right elbow.

precautions

● The rear shoulder is a very small muscle and it is easily strained or torn while being stretched, so perform this stretch very carefully.

● Make sure no tension is left in the relaxed arm. If any tension is still present, this signifies that a contraction is being performed, and such a contraction will usually involve the rear shoulder at some point—the very area you are trying to relax completely in order to stretch it.

rear upper arm stretch

benefits: This stretches your rear upper arm muscles and, as a side benefit, also stretches the sides of the upper back.

1 Stand with your bottom pushed out just a little (to minimize any forward rotation of the hips).

precautions

● Do not perform this stretch while moving around or walking, for two key reasons:
● The fact that both elbows are well away from your center of gravity (2 in. above your navel) makes your body weight a greater load for the lower back. This therefore means that the stability achieved by standing still is needed to ensure that tiny undetected micro tears in the lower back muscles are avoided as much as possible.
● Moving or walking also destabilizes the solidarity in your lower body that you have intentionally created (by pushing out your bottom) for the stretch happening in your upper body.

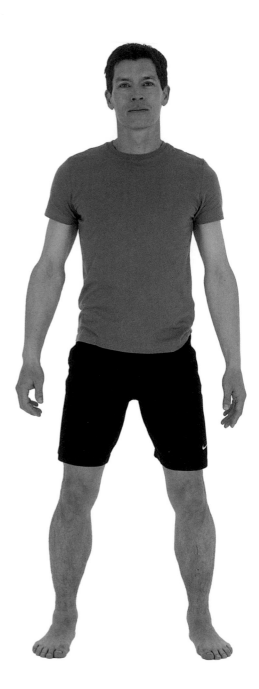

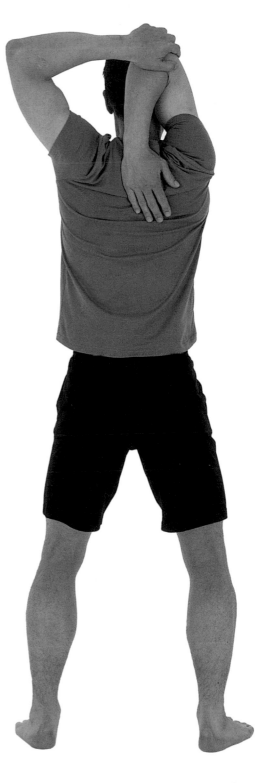

2 Take your arms overhead, and hold the elbow of one arm with the hand of the other. Now gently pull the elbow behind your head to enact a stretch in the rear upper arm. Hold the AA for a minimum of 30 seconds.

3 Repeat this stretch on the other arm.

trapezius stretch

benefits: If you suffer from headaches or any form of tension in your shoulder area, this particular stretch for the traps could be your salvation.

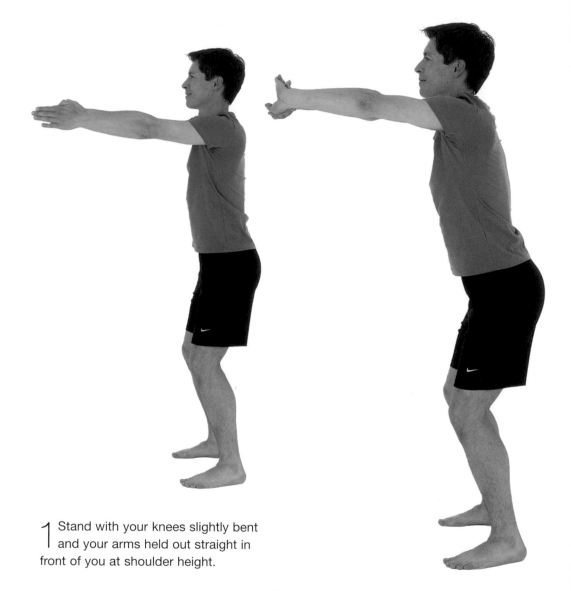

1 Stand with your knees slightly bent and your arms held out straight in front of you at shoulder height.

2 Interlace your fingers together, with your palms facing away from you. Gently push away with your palms until you feel a reasonably comfortable pressure against the fingers.

● The trapezius ("traps") is a big muscle that goes into the base of your skull at the back of your head, and although its size runs a good way down your upper middle back, it makes up a sizable portion of your shoulders on either side of your neck. Strictly speaking, there is more trapezius on your back than on your shoulders, but as the most effective stretches for it are felt at the shoulders, it is included in this shoulder section.

● The trapezius is widely responsible for many tension headaches, which is why massaging your shoulders on either side of your neck can help ease the discomfort.

● The upper arms are responsible for activity at the shoulders and back. When you hold something in your hands, such as a shovel in the garden, or pull on a rope, you feel tired in the shoulders. It is the actions of the upper arms that are dominantly responsible for the fatigue that you experienced.

● The elbows are the nearest real work point for your traps at the shoulders, and using your elbows can tense the trapezius, making it tight. For example, if you lean on your elbows for extended periods of time, or drive for some hours (when your arms are bent, but the upper arms are usually a little out from the body and slightly lifted), you will often develop a headache or some stiffness in your shoulders.

precautions

● Do not push your interlaced fingers too far away from you at the beginning of this technique. Bending the fingers to an uncomfortable degree is completely unnecessary, as it is the focused and careful rounding of the shoulders forward that is the essence of success here.

3 Slowly round your shoulders forward until you feel the AA sensation across them and on either side of your neck. Hold the AA for a minimum of 30 seconds.

deltoid stretch

benefits: This is a stretch for the shoulder muscles called the deltoids, which lie at the very outside of your shoulder. They interact with your trapezius in all shoulder work, so if you combine this stretch with your trapezius stretch after a long drive or working day, you should certainly be less stressed and more relaxed at the end.

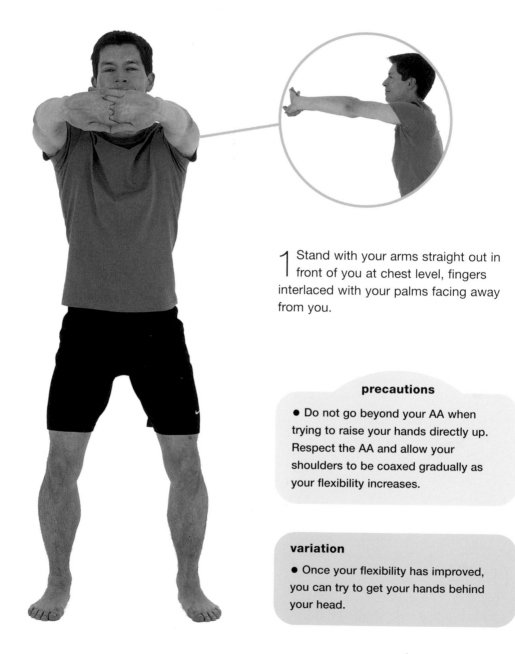

1 Stand with your arms straight out in front of you at chest level, fingers interlaced with your palms facing away from you.

precautions

● Do not go beyond your AA when trying to raise your hands directly up. Respect the AA and allow your shoulders to be coaxed gradually as your flexibility increases.

variation

● Once your flexibility has improved, you can try to get your hands behind your head.

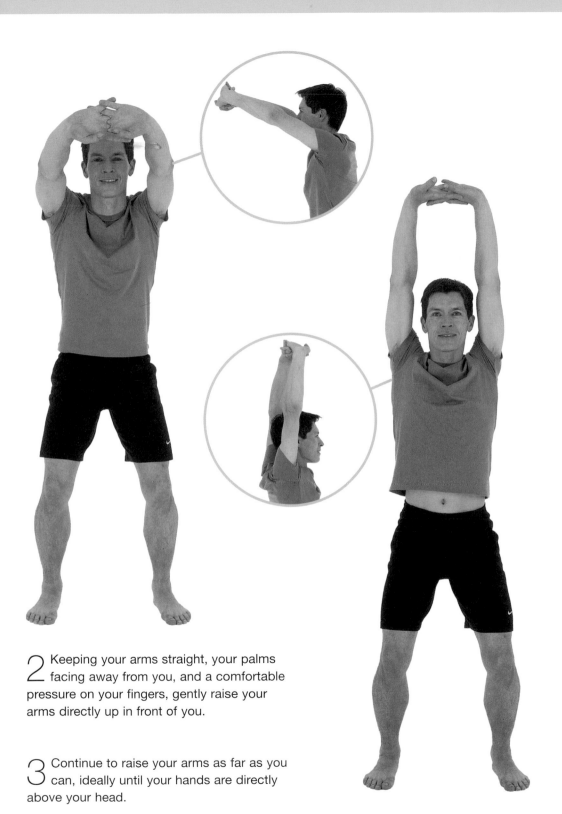

2 Keeping your arms straight, your palms facing away from you, and a comfortable pressure on your fingers, gently raise your arms directly up in front of you.

3 Continue to raise your arms as far as you can, ideally until your hands are directly above your head.

front upper arm stretch

benefits: The front upper arm incorporates a number of muscle groups, not just the bicep. Greater flexibility in this area enables a person to draw the arm back through a greater range of motion and consequently, enables more powerful movements on the return journey.

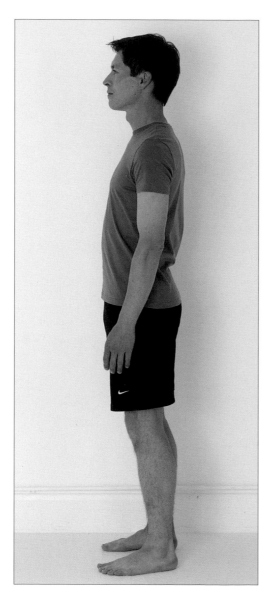

1 Position yourself very near a wall or a doorframe. Stand facing forward, with your arms hanging loosely at your sides and your legs slightly bent at the knees.

tip

The higher you place your fist, the earlier you will get to your AA, so be careful as you step forward and as you turn your torso. In both cases, the joint articulations of the front shoulders are stretched, which is not a bad thing, but just keep an eye on how much you are stretching that area. Eventually, as you get to know your body better, you can adjust the position to target your stretch focus more acutely on the front upper arm.

variation

● If you want to include your chest more in this stretch, then cup your fingers, with your palms flat, and "hook" onto the corner of the wall. This will, however, give much less stretch to your shoulder.

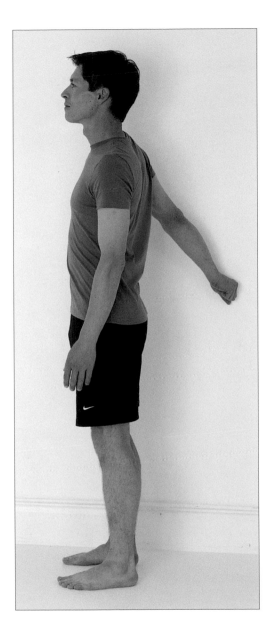

● The front upper arm muscle is one of the smallest and least significant of our muscles. It has only two parts as compared to the rear upper arm muscle, which has three, so in theory, the back of your upper arm is potentially more capable than your front when you consider the balance of total power available to you in the arms. Nevertheless, its flexibility is an integral part of your whole body flexibility.

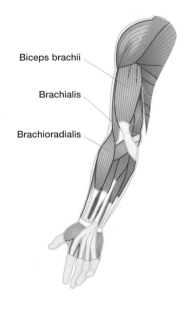

Biceps brachii

Brachialis

Brachioradialis

2 Make a gentle fist with your right hand, and place it against the wall with the index finger/thumb side of the fist in contact with it. Gently move a little sideways, away from your fist, until your right arm is comfortably straight.

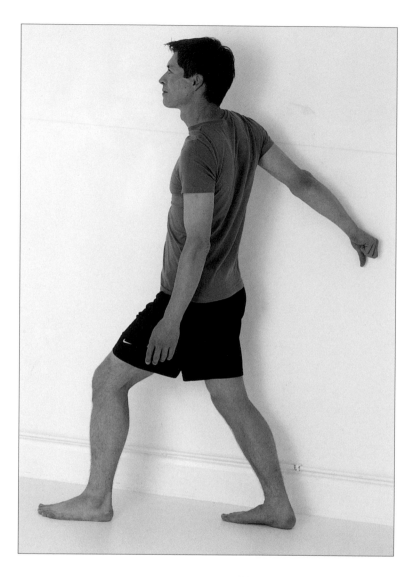

3 Once in this position, take a small step forward with your left foot, making absolutely sure both your legs have a very slight bend at the knees.

precautions

● Do not keep your legs straight when you turn, or you will twist your legs and put a high degree of stress on your knees. Just a slight bend to the knee will counteract this problem very well, as it automatically locks your pelvis in a forward-facing position a little more and in many physiques can even make the degree of rotation necessary to reach the AA a little less.

4 Very gently rotate your torso and attempt to look over your left shoulder. This will stretch the bicep of the right arm very efficiently and improve the flexibility of the forearm as well. Note that the height at which you place your fist radically affects your front shoulder and also the time it will take for you to reach your AA. Always start with your fist low on the wall and work your way carefully up, ensuring you stay below any sharp front shoulder sensation.

5 Hold the AA for a minimum of 30 seconds, then repeat with the other arm.

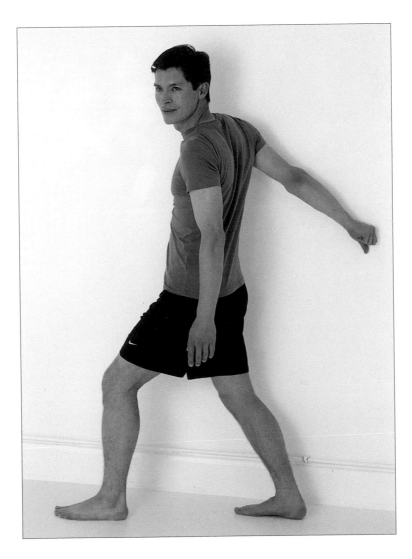

chest stretches

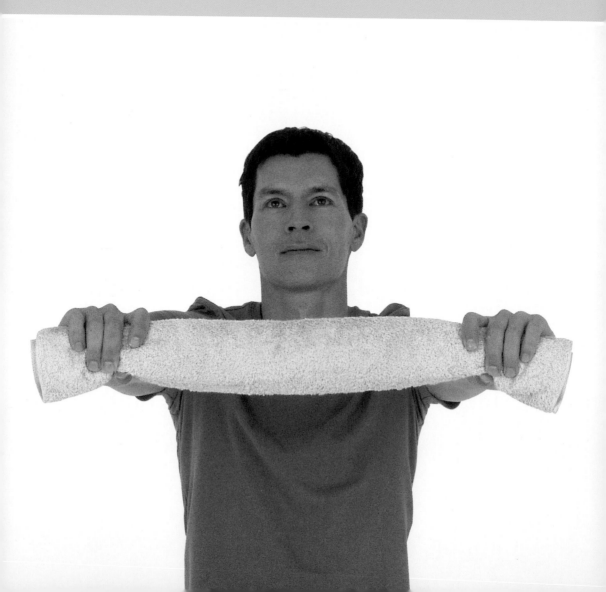

- the bow
- upper chest stretch

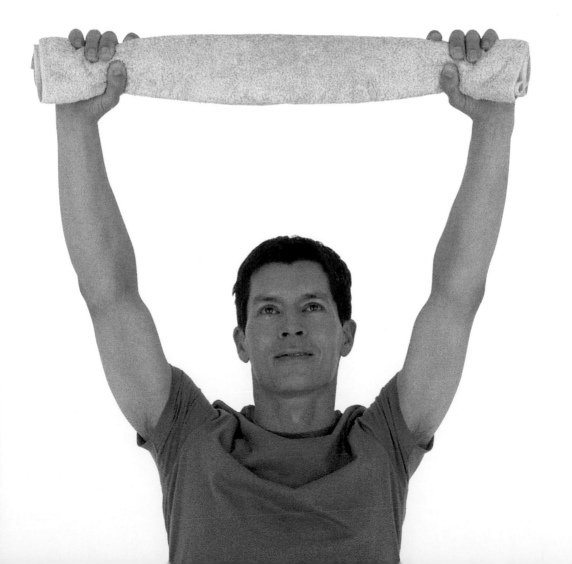

the bow

benefits: One of the advantages of a mobile and flexible chest area is a better and more efficient intake of air into the lungs. The muscles between your ribs (intercostals) become more capable in expansion and contraction. At the same time, the increased flexibility of the chest muscles (pectorals) aids the entire process.

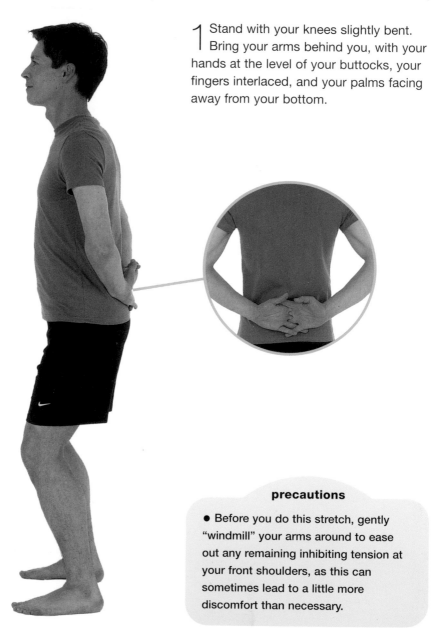

1 Stand with your knees slightly bent. Bring your arms behind you, with your hands at the level of your buttocks, your fingers interlaced, and your palms facing away from your bottom.

precautions

● Before you do this stretch, gently "windmill" your arms around to ease out any remaining inhibiting tension at your front shoulders, as this can sometimes lead to a little more discomfort than necessary.

2 Now straighten your arms, gently pushing out your chest while carefully easing your elbows toward each other.

tip

Stretches in the front shoulders, biceps, and forearms are a side benefit of this technique, but do not lose sight of the fact that it is the chest you are predominantly trying to stretch here.

variation

● Women usually have less substance across their backs than men, and so they may need a developmental measure to enable them to feel the AA. This is achieved by initially turning the palms to face away from the body. Then, once the elbows have been eased closer to each other, the hands can be taken back and away from the body until the AA is felt.

upper chest stretch

benefits: A supple and flexible upper chest area allows greater movement by the arms anywhere above parallel. Exercising this area can also prevent kyphosis, a round-shouldered posture that can cause backache.

1 Stand comfortably balanced, slightly bent at the knees, with the buttocks pushed out gently a little way behind you. Hold a rolled-up towel with a palms-down grip at full arm's length away from you at waist level. Hands should be a little wider than shoulder-width apart, ensuring the towel remains straight by exerting a constant, gentle pull. Your line of vision should be directly forward.

precautions

● Never bring the towel to the overhead position and, without letting go, take it straight through, up, and over, and down to the position near your buttocks. This will traumatise your shoulder articulations.

2 Keeping the gentle pull and arms straight, raise the towel upward until it is directly overhead or, if you're very flexible, slightly behind your head.

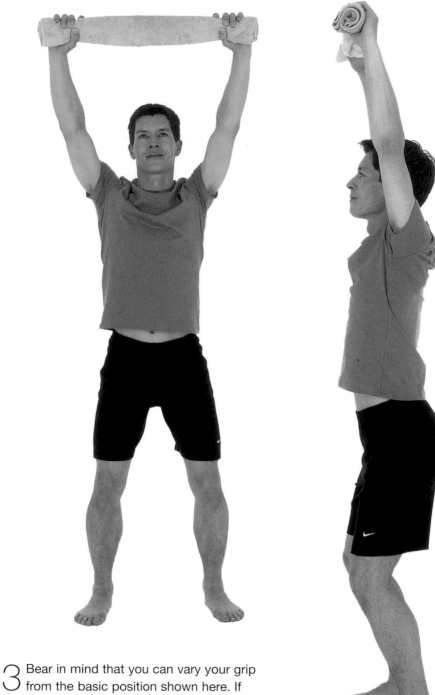

3 Bear in mind that you can vary your grip
  from the basic position shown here. If
you find that adopting a narrower grip
produces a more efficient AA sensation in the
chest area, then by all means do so.

variation

● You can also begin this stretch approach with the towel behind you (see right). The arms are still kept straight to ensure the towel remains rigid. Raise the arms up behind you until you feel the AA in the chest. Usually, this rear approach will make the AA happen sooner, but front or back, the choice is yours.

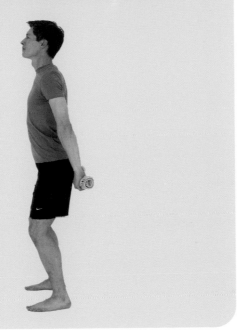

fact file

● Make sure you never look down when performing this stretch. Always look comfortably up, otherwise the excessive slackening of the neck muscles will decrease the efficency of the technique. Consequently, this decrease would reduce the productive stretch in the area above the collar bone around which the chest muscles are anchored before spreading down and out over the rib cage. If the neck muscles are being stretched up and back at the same time as the shoulders are being drawn back, a good upper chest stretch is much more achievable.

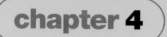

chapter 4

back stretches

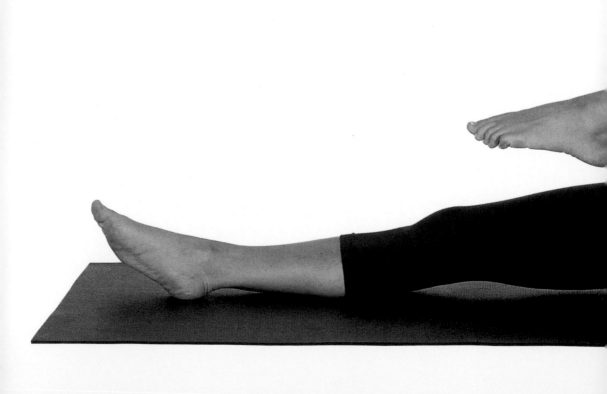

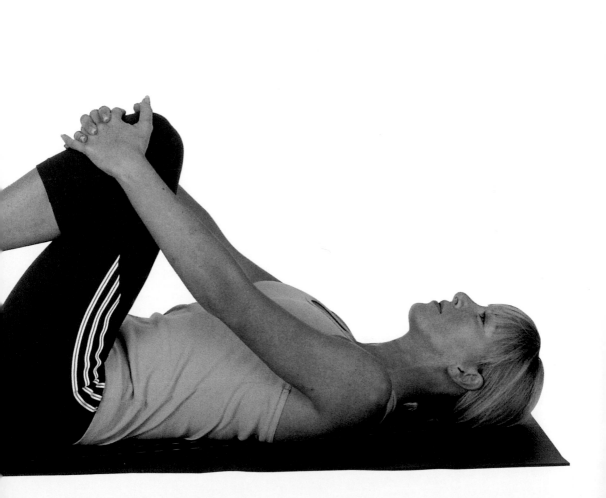

- gluteal tightening
- prone and supine hands
- the long reach
- knee to chest stretch

- lying trunk twists
- back stretch
- the fetal position
- the worshipper

gluteal tightening

benefits: This exercise relieves the tension in your lower back.

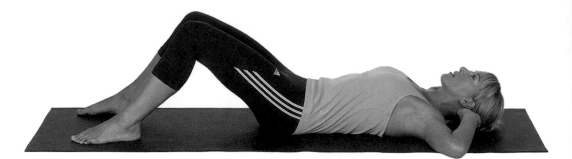

1 Lie on your back with your head resting on your hands. Your knees should be comfortably bent, with both feet firmly flat on the floor.

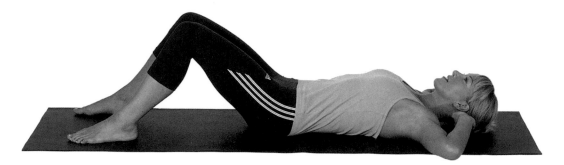

2 Tighten the muscles of your bottom (gluteals) while simultaneously tightening your abdominal muscles. This will automatically flatten your lower back for you.

tip

The more you perform this action, the more your tightening/contractile power will grow. Within weeks, you will be able to achieve a contraction that is way beyond your initial maximum capability.

3 Sustain the tightening for at least 30 seconds, then release the tightened muscles gently to avoid jerking them.

tip

The success of the contraction is achieved by maintaining it at a constant level. If you try to maintain the maximum tightening you can achieve, you will in fact be performing a series of minor contractions on and off the actual maximum point itself. Aim instead for what you perceive to be around 85 percent of your maximum. This will still be a strong enough tightening for your purpose, and you are far more likely to be able to maintain that level constantly.

fact file

● The core muscles, as seen here, are essential to good posture and support for the body. With an exercise such as gluteal tightening, there is very little obvious movement because you are exercising muscles deep in the body. But these exercises are crucial to your general health and fitness—particularly as you get older or after childbirth.

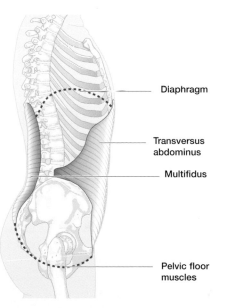

Diaphragm

Transversus abdominus

Multifidus

Pelvic floor muscles

prone and supine hands

benefits: Prone is palms down and supine is palms up. One of the great advantages of this stretch is its opportunity for the individual to focus more on one side of the body that might be less flexible or tighter than the other.

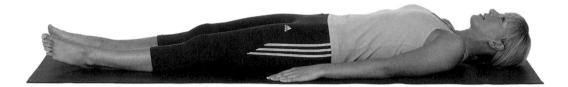

1 Lie on your back with your hands by your sides, palms face down. This is known as a prone hand position.

fact file

● When one side of the back is less flexible than the other, it can cause problems. One of these is scoliosis, where a sideways tilt of the torso occurs because of a curve in the spine. Unsuspecting mothers often encourage such a scenario by balancing their baby on one hip thrust out to the side as they hold conversations. Done repeatedly, this often has a negative effect on the spine.

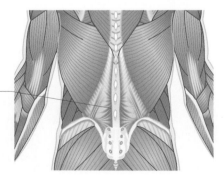

Erector Spinae
(lumbar spine)

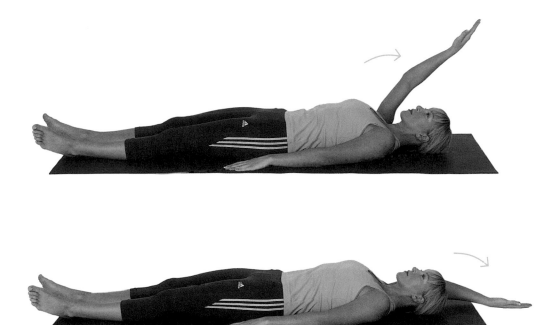

2 Move your right arm above your head and onto the floor behind you with your palm facing up. This is known as a supine hand position.

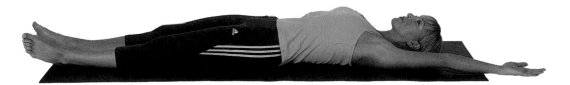

3 Do this for a minimum of 30 seconds, then change arms.

precautions

● Do not force the back of the hand with the palm facing up down to the floor—just feel the stretch in your upper back (and also to a greater or lesser degree to your shoulders) to the AA.

the long reach

benefits: This is probably the simplest stretch there is, and, as a result, it is often considerably underrated. Applied gently and slowly, it is suitable for anyone with very restricted mobility and flexibility levels.

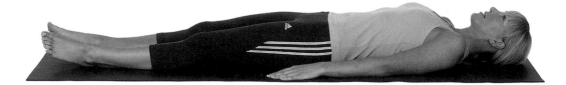

1 Lie on your back, extend your arms overhead with your palms facing upward, and straighten your legs out completely.

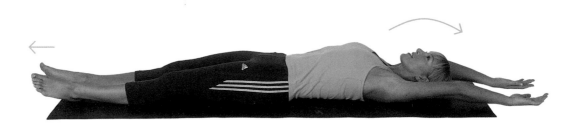

2 Reach out in opposite directions with your arms and legs as far as you comfortably can to the AA, ensuring you stretch your fingers out and point your toes.

3 Sustain the stretch for a minimum of 30 seconds, then move directly into the knee to chest stretch (see opposite).

knee to chest stretch

benefits: Another exercise that allows you to concentrate on one side of the body. This is of particular benefit to anyone who regularly uses one side of the body, such as a long jumper who has a "take off" leg or a gardener who is often digging.

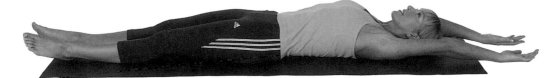

1 Start in step 3 position of the long reach (see opposite).

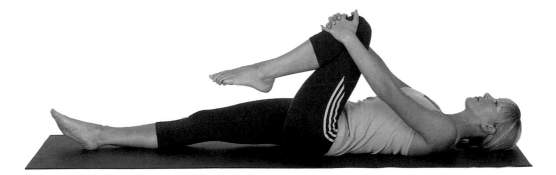

2 Pull your left leg toward your chest. Try to keep the back of your head on the floor throughout, and keep your lower back as flat as possible, as long as you can manage this without strain. Hold that position for a minimum of 30 seconds, before repeating it with the other leg.

tip

Owing to the position of your thigh against the rib cage and stomach in step 2, you may find that you will be breathing a little more shallowly and in slightly shorter intervals than normal, but as long as you are comfortable, this is fine.

3 Finish the stretch by pulling both knees to your chest (the closer they are to your chest at the front, the greater the stretch in the back) and relaxing again in the AA for a minimum of 30 seconds.

lying trunk twists

benefits: This exercise stretches and firms the muscles over the sciatic nerve, which travels down the leg and foot from the lower spinal area. This minimizes any unnecessary pressure on this nerve.

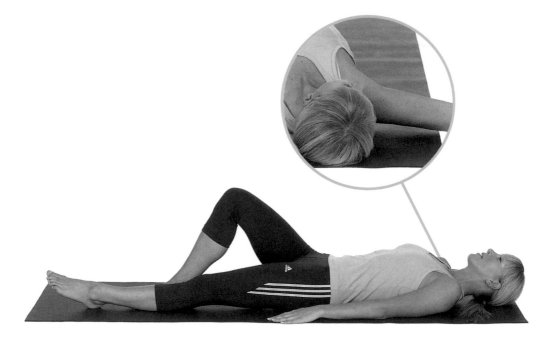

1 Lie on your back on the floor and extend your right arm (with your palm down) directly out at 90 degrees to your upper body.

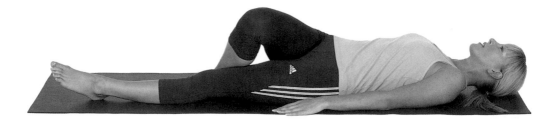

2 Now bend your right leg at 90 degrees also, and take it across your body to the left.

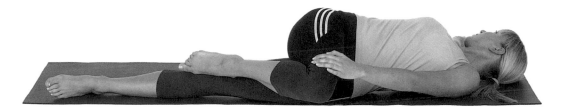

3 With your head resting on the floor, turn to look to your right.

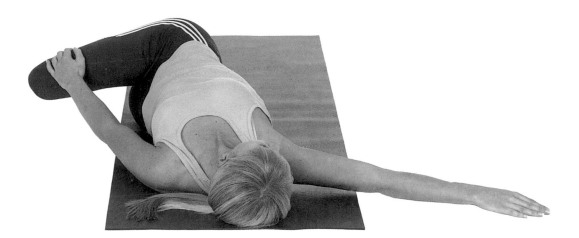

4 Rest your left hand just above your right knee and use it to pull your right leg down toward the floor, keeping your feet and ankles as relaxed as possible. Try to keep your shoulders flat on the floor to receive the full benefit of the stretch. Hold for a minimum for 30 seconds.

5 Reverse the position to apply the same flexibility training to the left-hand side of your back.

back stretch

benefits: A good stretch for anyone on the move, who needs to stretch out. This stretches and relaxes your spinal muscles.

1 Stand with your feet slightly apart. With the knees bent, push your bottom out behind you just a little.

2 Bend forward from the waist, with shoulders rounded and hands on knees, and lower yourself gently down—keeping close to the front of your body as you do—until you feel the stretch in your back.

tip

Placing your hands on your knees or lower leg and keeping your bottom gently pushed out help maximize the stretch. They also allow you to use your hands to control the descent and stop at the AA, when this gentle forward flop has taken you to the right flexibility point.

the fetal position

benefits: This stretch, which eases both the sides and the lower area of the back, is the ultimate calming-down strategy. It is simple to perform and is the most naturally restful position there is for the human body, mimicking our time in the womb.

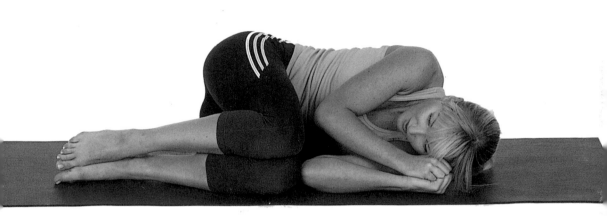

1 Lie on your side.

2 Draw your legs up and rest your head on your hands. Concentrate on relaxing all the muscles in your body, allowing your feet, hands, and facial muscles to relax. Close your eyes and breathe naturally. This position follows the natural contours of the body and is probably the most relaxed position in existence.

the worshipper

benefits: This stretch opens up the muscles across the back, from lower to upper and beneath the shoulder blades. It effectively releases tension in the all-important postural support muscles—the muscles that work hard at keeping you upright all day.

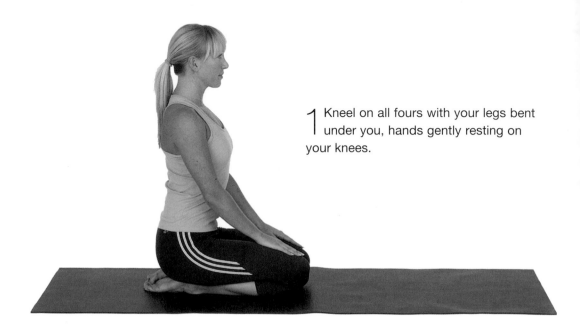

1 Kneel on all fours with your legs bent under you, hands gently resting on your knees.

tips

- Exhaling before you make the descent with your torso will decrease the sense of air retention in the midsection, and the feeling of "emptying" you experience will make the descent that much more efficient.
- If you perform this stretch on a rug, you can hold onto the edge of the rug and pull yourself further forward.
- Having your thighs quite wide apart will help you lower your entire body to the floor.

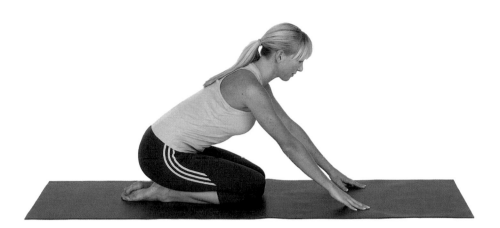

2 Gently ease down and backward with your torso, extending your arms straight out in front of you, until you get as much as you can of the underside of both your arms and chest on the floor. Get your face down as close as you can to the floor itself, as though you were prostrating yourself on a prayer mat.

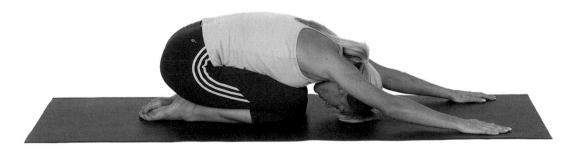

variation

● Small, subtle movements to each side with your hips can change the focus of the stretch. The way your body will react to this variation will be unique to your own physiology.

3 Once you are at the AA in the back and shoulders, hold for a minimum of 30 seconds.

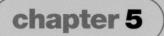

chapter 5
abdominal stretches

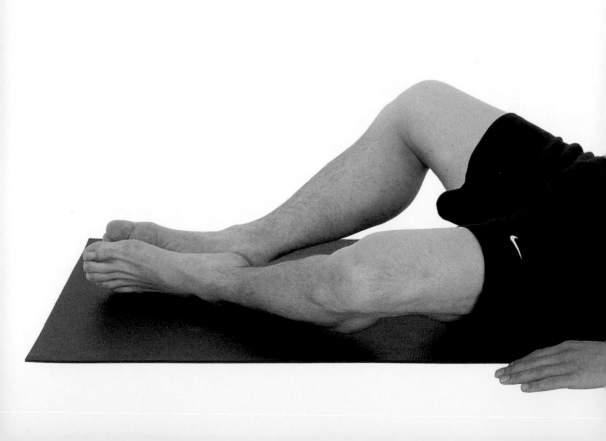

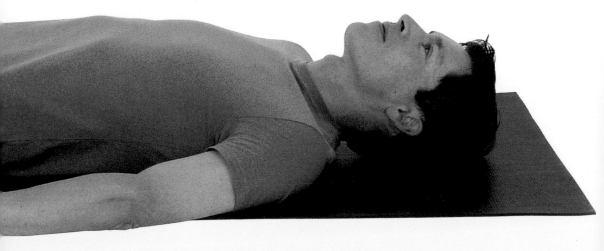

cobra stretch

benefits: This is an outstanding abdominal stretch that is highly effective and works for the vast majority of people even at a very basic postural level. It is the only progressive abdominal stretch you will ever need.

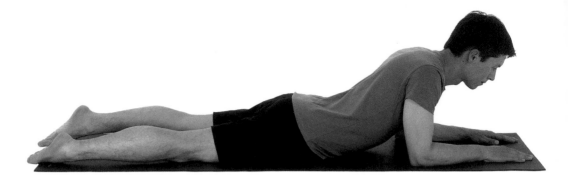

1 Lie face down on the floor. Bend your arms and support yourself on your elbows with the palms of your hands face down on the floor.

2 Place your elbows a little forward of your torso. Looking straight ahead, firmly press down flat with the palms of your hands and the underside of your forearms, until you establish a "grip" on the floor.

precautions

● Never straighten your arms during the execution of this technique, as you can hyperextend the lower back, putting pressure on the intervertebral discs and causing injury.

3 Now, make the motion of drawing your arms back along the floor, but allow the grip you have established to stop you from actually moving. You will remain constantly in a restricted "draw back" action that never results in you actually allowing your hands or elbows to move back at all. This has already begun to stretch your abdominal muscles and also the very important muscles between your ribs (intercostals), which are an integral element in making your abdominal area more flexible.

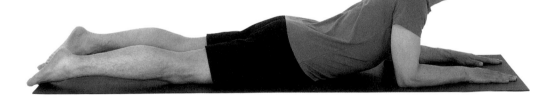

4 Keeping the palm-to-elbow "draw back" in motion, gently add to the growing stretch feel by pushing your chest out. It might not feel as though you are able to push it out a great deal at all in this floor position, but you will achieve further graduated expansion of your rib cage here, to add to the final stretch application.

5 Very slowly, gently let your head tilt directly back and try to look up at the ceiling. The tilt of the head is a carefully administered move, so be sure to take it very carefully and slowly, as a quick jerk back will certainly strain your neck. As your head travels back, you should become aware of the AA happening. If it doesn't happen straight away, push your chest out a little more.

cobra stretch variation

benefits: These adjustments to the basic cobra allow you to stretch the sides of your abdominal muscles, too.

1 Apply the same initial posture: palms-to-elbow "draw back" and chest out.

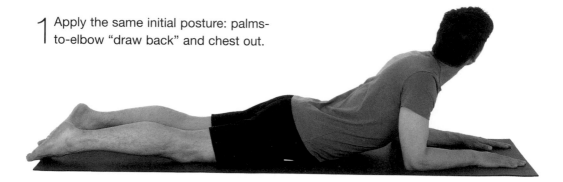

2 If you want to stretch the right-hand side of your abdominal muscles, look up at the ceiling again and hold the AA for a minimum of 30 seconds. Then, gently and deliberately turn your head to look to your upper left. Hold for a minimum of 30 seconds.

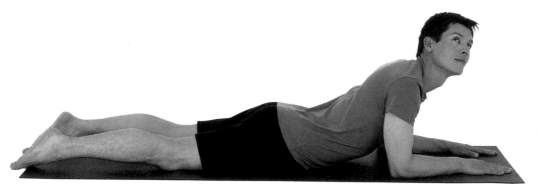

precautions

● Never straighten your arms: their bent position and the further-forward position of the elbows are what protect your back.

3 If you want to stretch the left-hand side of your abdominal muscles, return to the AA, hold, and then turn your head slowly and deliberately to look to your upper right, holding at the AA again.

abdominal stretch I

benefits: This is particularly effective as a pre-natal abdominal stretch. Pay careful attention to bending the knee gently and a sensible non-pressurized sensation will be felt in the lower back (lumbar-sacral area).

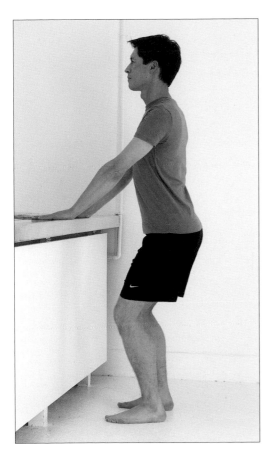

1 Stand facing a waist-high surface, such as a table, windowsill, or automobile hood. Place your feet in an easy stance, legs slightly bent at the knees, and your bottom pushed out very gently behind you. Gently place the palms of your hands on the surface, shoulder-width apart.

2 Very carefully move back a fraction until your arms are absolutely straight, remembering to keep your legs very slightly bent at the knees and your bottom slightly out behind you. Keep your line of vision directly forward.

3 Once you are in this position, there will be a sensation of the shoulders rounding forward very slightly and it is that slight bending of your knees and the bottom out behind you that protects you from even the slightest lower back trauma while you perform this stretch. There may already be, even at this stage, a feeling of stretch around the rib cage and abdominals, which signals that you will not have to develop this much further to attain your AA.

4 Very gently, making sure you keep your arms completely straight, apply pressure down through your palms onto the surface of the table. Once you are sustaining this moderate pressure through your palms, initiate a "draw back" action (see cobra stretch), which merely grips the table surface. The palms will not move, as the movement toward you is halted by the downward pressure.

precautions

● You can push your bottom out a little more or increase the bend at the knees if required for the AA to be achieved. However, when bending further at the knees, remember to keep your bottom pushed gently out behind you to ensure the safety of your knees.
● If you increase the thrust in your chest, pay attention to your lower back. This is an abdominal stretch and you should not be feeling the stretch more in your lower back than in your stomach and around your rib cage. If you are feeling this, try bending at the knees a little more or moving a little further from the surface.
● Do not allow your arms to bend at any point in the stretch technique.
● Do not stop applying the sustained down and backward pressure of your palms on the surface.

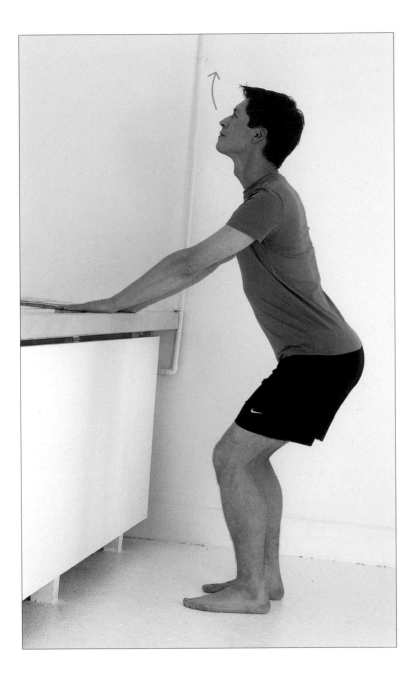

5 Now, gently push your chest out, lift your head, and gradually look directly up and back. Move your head slowly and carefully to avoid getting a crick in your neck. You should have a slow awareness of the AA setting in. Hold for 30 seconds.

abdominal stretch II

benefits: Although this stretch is often referred to as a groin stretch, one of its greatest benefits is to render the lower inner abdominals (sometimes referred to as the inguinal area) more flexible. This stretch is particularly good for anyone with back problems, as the back is relaxed and never used directly.

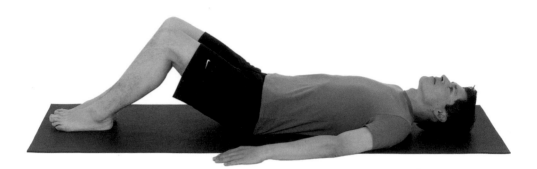

1 Lie on the floor on your back with your knees bent and your palms face down. You should feel no strain in the lower back.

fact file

• Flexibility in the inguinal area goes a long way to help prevent conditions such as hernias and inner thigh muscle tears and strains, which can occur when lifting heavy objects. It also protects against sudden unexpected thigh traumas, such as slipping and falling with the legs spread-eagled sideways or forward.
• Maintaining the squeeze in your buttocks naturally raises your pelvis off the floor. This action provides enough safe elevation to make the limb weight of your upper thighs descend further apart on either side of your pelvis. The weight of the thighs themselves increases the stretch effect. Placing the hands on the thighs and encouraging the process further (if you have not reached the AA by then) is the next step.

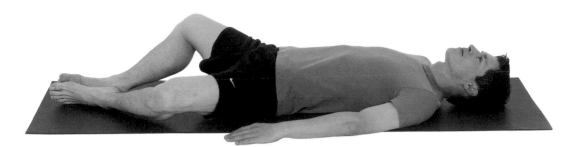

2 Carefully draw your legs up and, without forcing the position in any way, place the soles of your feet together, regardless of how far or close to the groin area your feet are to achieve this. At this point you may already be sensing a stretch effect in your inner upper thigh/lower abdominals, so proceed carefully and stop immediately you experience your own AA as we progress through the developmental adjustments. This is as far as you will need to go.

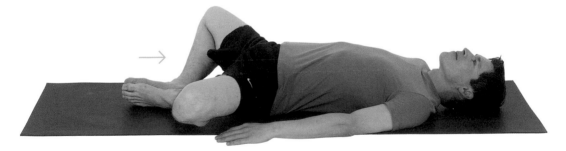

3 Once the soles of your feet are symmetrically together, very gently draw your knees up toward you until you feel the stretch response beginning in your groin/lower stomach muscles. Do not arch your back off the floor, and keep your head on the floor, too, with your neck and shoulders relaxed. Now, squeeze your buttocks and hold that contraction. If you prefer, you can very gently push down on the inner thighs with your hands until you reach your AA. Your back and head must remain on the floor.

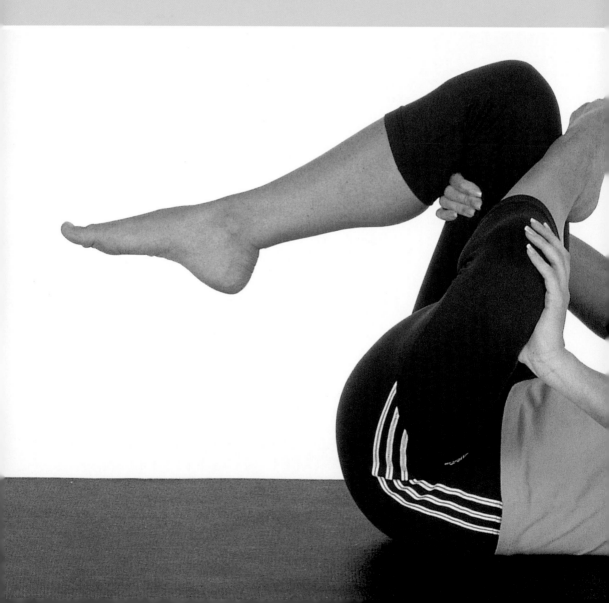

ankle, feet, and leg stretches

hamstring stretch I

benefits: This first in a series of three stretches for the rear upper thigh is an excellent way of stretching your hamstring muscles, particularly the end of them, which insert behind your knees in a generally less accessible area.

1 With the base of your spine supported against a wall, chair, or sofa, sit upright with both legs stretched out.

2 Gently draw the toes on both feet back toward your shins until you just feel an awareness in your front lower legs.

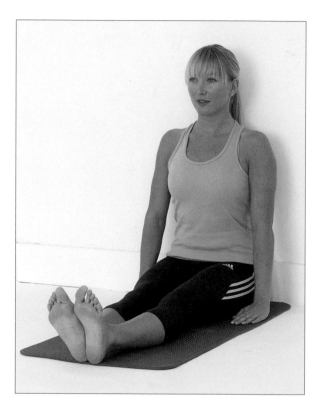

tip

The rear upper thigh also contains your calf muscles, and this exercise will stretch those muscles, too.

precautions

● Do not neglect to draw your toes back. This action is what stretches the lower hamstring, and without it you will put pressure on your lower back, possibly causing subclinical micro-trauma there. It is for this reason that this exercise should always be done with your spine supported.

● Do not perform this stretch using a towel or scarf wrapped around your foot in order to pull on your calf muscles manually while you lean forward. This tends to place too much focus on the calf muscles themselves, and you will probably reach your AA before thoroughly stretching your hamstrings.

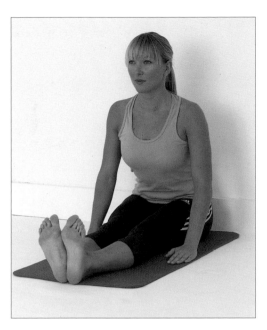

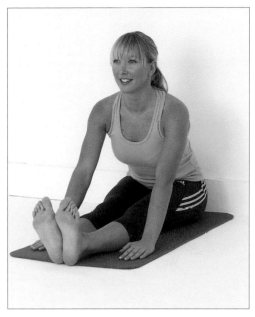

3 Maintain this gentle toes-drawn-back position, then, supporting yourself on your hands, gently "walk" your hands down the outside of your thighs until you reach the AA in your rear upper thighs. Hold for a minimum of 30 seconds.

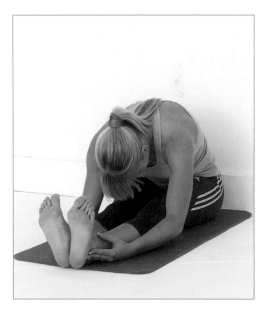

fact file

● Tight hamstrings are a cause of many knock-on problems elsewhere in the body. If hamstrings are excessively tight, they can cause lower back problems, front thigh and knee problems, and mid/rear shoulder and neck problems.

hamstring stretch II

benefits: This will provide a more challenging stretch than stretch I if you are quite loose and flexible. However, ensure you are confident of your flexibility before attempting this stronger stretch.

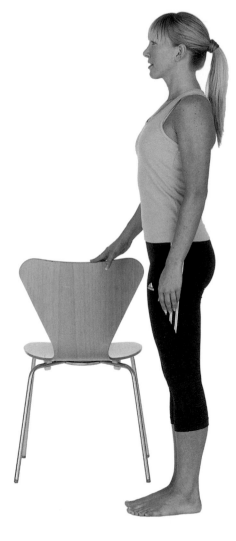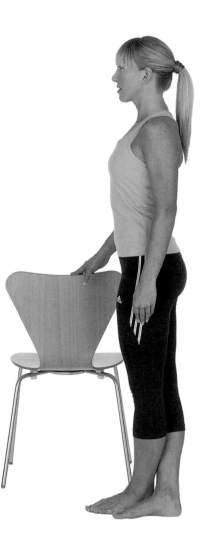

1 Stand in front of a chair, cross your left
  foot over your right, and rest your
hand or elbow (depending on how flexible
you already are in your back and
hamstrings) on the back of the seat.

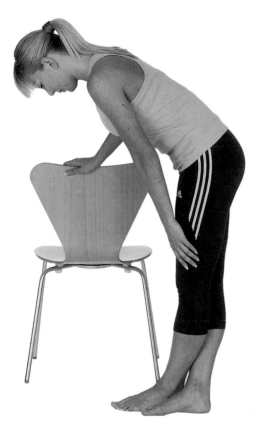

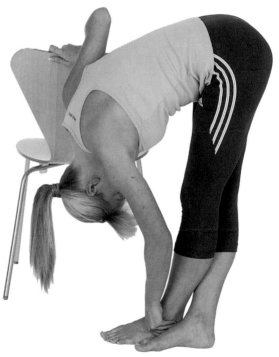

2 Push your bottom out gently and, keeping your left leg comfortably bent and your right leg as straight as possible, lower yourself gently forward and down so that your head moves nearer the seat of the chair. Lower your torso down toward the thighs.

precautions

● For the sake of total control and because of the involvement of the ligaments of the lower spine, perform this stretch near a support such as a chair, sofa, or fence post.

3 You will find that comparatively little descent is required before you reach your AA in the rear of your upper right leg. Hold the AA for a minimum of 30 seconds, then push against the chair to get upright again.

4 Repeat the stretch, crossing your right foot over your left.

hamstring stretch III

benefits: You will need to move very little to reach your AA in this stretch. The fact that, unusually for a hamstring stretch, both your legs are straight means that less pressure is placed on the supporting leg.

1 Stand with your legs straight and your left foot placed on a chair. Rest your right hand on the back of the chair.

variation

● Once you can perform this stretch easily and safely, you will not need to hold onto anything, and can instead place both hands on the front thigh of the limb being stretched. This centralizes the entire torso weight and the extra pressure of the weight of our hands pressing down increases the hamstring stretch.

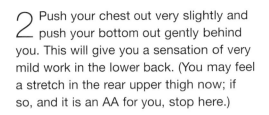

2 Push your chest out very slightly and push your bottom out gently behind you. This will give you a sensation of very mild work in the lower back. (You may feel a stretch in the rear upper thigh now; if so, and it is an AA for you, stop here.)

3 Choose something directly in front of you at eye level to focus on, and lock your eyes on it. Now, draw the toes of your left foot very gently toward your shin, until you have a sensation along the upper calf and rear upper thigh (usually more behind the knee at this stage).

4 Then, gently and very slowly lean forward and down, while keeping your eyes firmly on your chosen focus point. Hold at the AA for a minimum of 30 seconds. Repeat with your right leg on the chair.

lying front thigh stretch

benefits: This lying-down stretch increases the flexibility of the quadriceps (the large muscles in the front of the thigh).

1 Lie on your left side on the floor, with your elbow on the floor supporting your upper body weight.

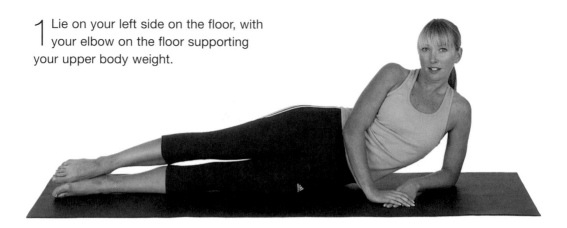

2 Bend your right leg at the knee and bring it back, then clasp the foot with your right hand.

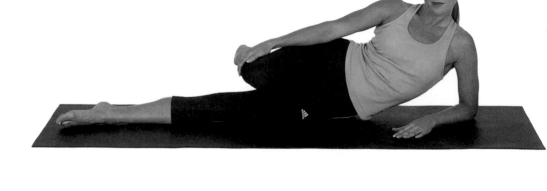

3 Gently draw your leg back until you feel the stretch in the front thigh, until you reach the AA.

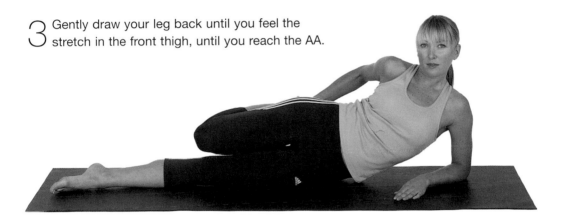

4 Hold for a minimum of 30 seconds, then repeat lying on your right side.

precautions

● Never perform this stretch in a standing position.

standing front thigh stretch

benefits: This stretch is good when you have limited space or outside when the weather is less than hospitable with soaking wet ground.

1 Stand, holding onto a support such as a chair back or countertop. Your knees should be soft, and your arms relaxed. Look straight ahead.

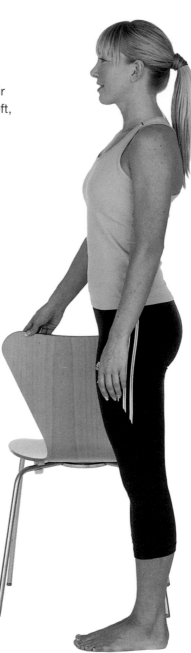

precautions

● Do not vary this exercise by holding a foot with the same-side arm (i.e., right hand holding your right foot). If you do this, your entire torso weight will be significantly displaced to one side, placing the spinal column in a position called "scoliosis" (a pronounced sideways angle to the spine that can lead to chronic back problems).

2 Gently draw your right leg back behind you until you reach the AA, and hold this for a minimum of 30 seconds. Then reach down behind you with your left hand, while bending your right leg and bringing your foot up behind you so you can grab it. Initially, you may have to bend your left leg a little to do this.

3 Repeat the stretch on the other side, lifting your left foot up and grabbing it with your right hand.

variation

● You can also perform this stretch lying down on your front. Some individuals will experience an added stretch across the outside of the thigh when in the lying posture.

inner thigh stretch

benefits: This technique stretches the inner thigh/groin muscles, the benefits of which can range from assisting the efficiency of the pelvic floor muscles to a more powerful sideways pass of the ball in soccer.

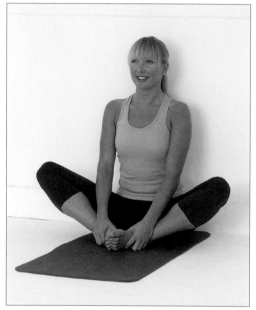

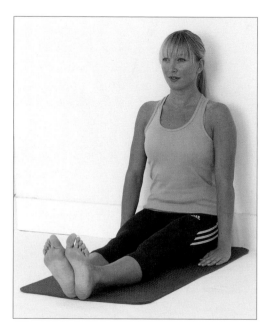

2 Bend your legs and draw the soles of your feet toward each other. This will cause the thighs to travel out and away from each other.

1 Sit on the floor with the base of your spine well supported against a wall or piece of securely anchored furniture.

precautions

● The inner thigh muscles are among the tightest and least stretched of all our muscle groups, and so need to be handled carefully. Overstretching them can cause painful groin strains and days, or even weeks, of uncomfortable immobility.
● Do not perform this stretch without a back support: the support is vital for preventing lower backache.

variation

● As you work on your flexibility, you will find that you are able to get your feet together and pull them much closer to your groin before you apply the downward pressure with your elbows or hands.

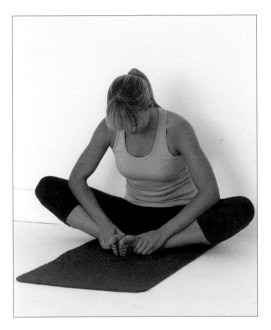

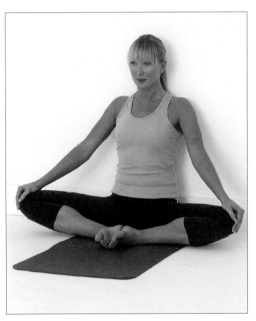

3 Once the soles of your feet are together (or very nearly if you are significantly inflexible), lean gently forward and hold your ankles (or just above them). As you lean, make sure you keep snuggling your lower back against your supportive surface to ensure your spine and pelvis never move too far away from it. Place your elbows on the inside of your knees and very, very gently push them out and down.

4 To add to the stretch, you can place your hands on the inside of your knees and then push down with them instead of your elbows until the AA is reached and hold for a minimum of 30 seconds.

ankle stretch

benefits: The gentle circular action of this stretch is probably the most all-round effective way of stretching and increasing the ankles' durable flexibility.

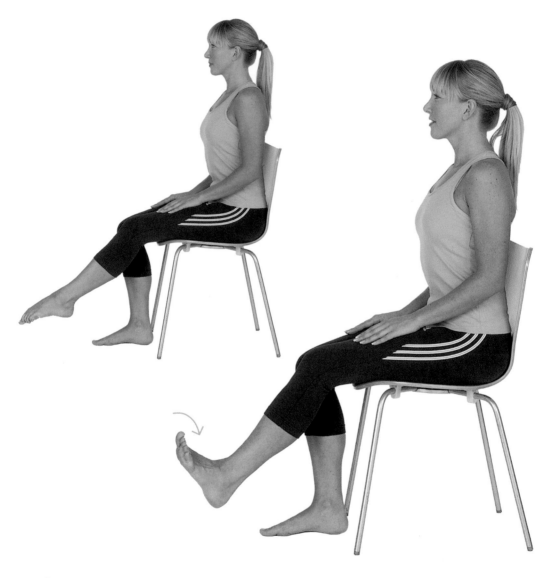

1 Sit on a chair, with your knees bent and feet flat on the ground, your hands resting gently on your thighs. Look straight ahead. Lift your left foot off the ground and begin to move it round in a clockwise direction.

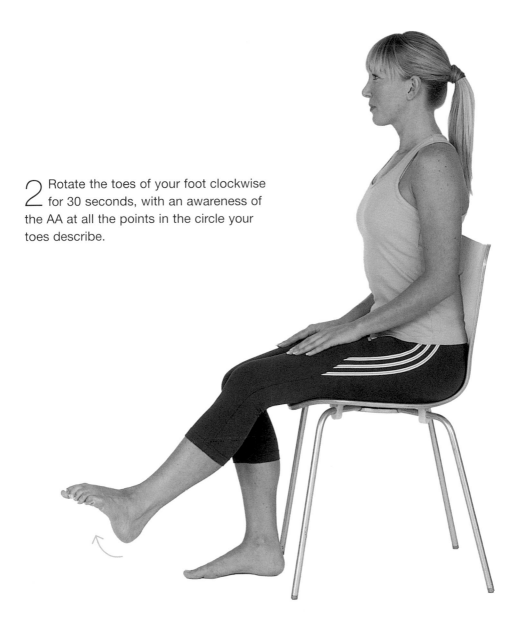

2 Rotate the toes of your foot clockwise for 30 seconds, with an awareness of the AA at all the points in the circle your toes describe.

precautions

● Do not force yourself to the very outer limits of the circle you are capable of creating. Stay a tiny fraction within it, as this will prevent any excessive tension in the calf and shin as you rotate.

3 Repeat in a counterclockwise movement for 30 seconds, then change to the other foot.

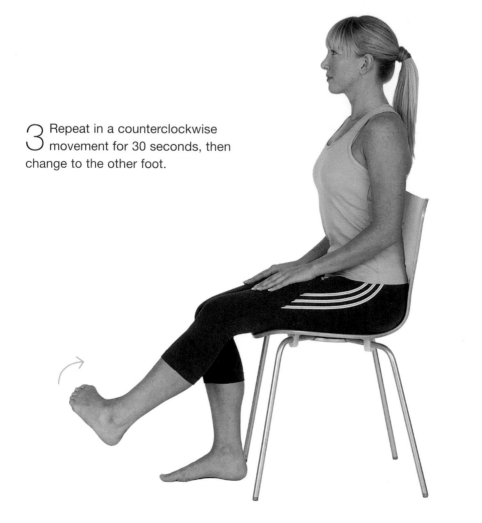

fact file

● The ankles are an important area to stretch, as they absorb a great deal of pressure and shock when the feet hit the ground in any activity. The outer ankle, which is slightly larger than its inner counterpart, is part of the shinbone and is consequently stronger and more solid than the inner ankle.

● Stretching the ankles in isolation presents some problems, as many of the stretches recommended cause significant tension in other muscles. For example, if the toes are pointed and held in that position, the lower end of the shin muscle, where it meets the upper structures of the ankle, will certainly get an effective stretch, but a palpable tension will be felt in the Achilles tendon and calf, possibly leading to a cramp in the lower calf.

gluteal stretch

benefits: This stretch will keep your buttocks very flexible and supple.

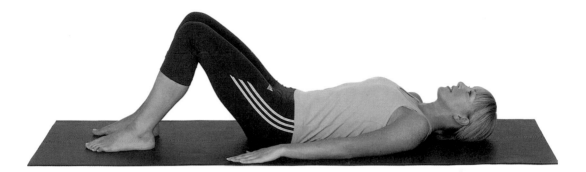

1 Lie on your back with your legs comfortably bent at the knees, and your feet a fairly good distance from your buttocks, to ensure an "open" angle at the knees.

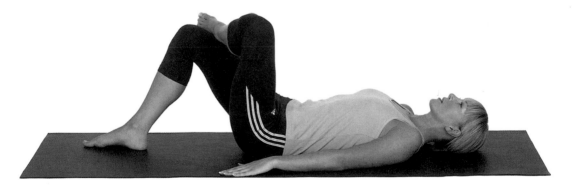

2 Place your left foot above the knee on your right thigh, taking the right knee out and away from your body as you do so. This position will already be placing a stretch on the left buttock, the degree of which depends on how flexible you are.

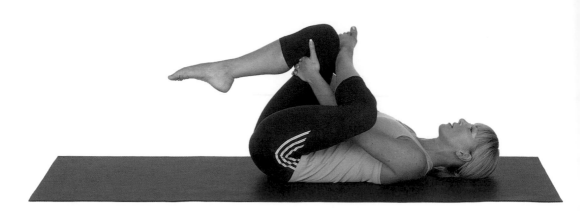

3 Development from this basic position to give greater flexibility can be achieved in four ways, but with them all, you really must retain an acute awareness of how the knee of the bent, buttock-stretching leg feels. Any really pronounced discomfort or actual pain is not acceptable, and in this case you should apply the AA principle to the knee area as well as the buttocks. The steps you can take, which should all be taken gently, by degree, are as follows:

4 Grab your right leg, hooking your fingers behind the thigh. Then draw the right leg back toward you.

precautions

● Avoid damaging your knees by combining a selection of the four approaches that suit your physical responses best.

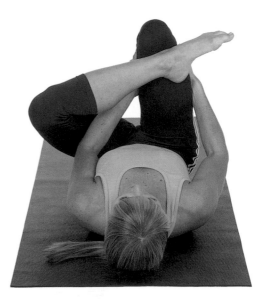

5 Move your left foot further to the right at the level of the right knee.

6 Push down on the inside of the left knee with your left hand.

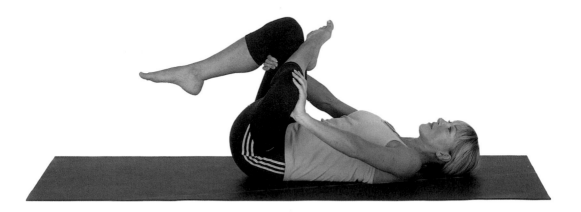

7 Finally, if you still feel that the AA in your buttock is capable of giving you greater range, sit up just enough to allow you to slip your hands around the back of your left thigh, interlacing your fingers behind it. Then very gently lean back and, if you can, rest your head on the floor

8 Repeat the stretch using the other leg.

fact file

● The gluteal muscles are the strongest muscles in the human body and are the foundation upon which your spinal muscles depend. If these muscles are inflexible and tight, they will impair the action of virtually every muscle in and around the pelvis. After the hamstrings, these are probably the most important group to keep supple.

lunge stretch

benefits: This very effective stretch, and one that is least traumatic on the knees, stretches the very upper part of the thigh muscles where they insert into your pelvis and the lower abdominal muscles (known as the hip flexors).

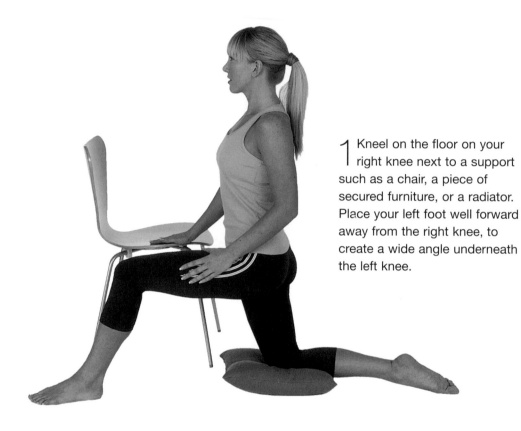

1 Kneel on the floor on your right knee next to a support such as a chair, a piece of secured furniture, or a radiator. Place your left foot well forward away from the right knee, to create a wide angle underneath the left knee.

tip

It is a good idea to use cushions to pad the knees when doing stretches of this nature, as often even the mildest pressure or discomfort at the knees can be detrimental to their safety.

precautions

● Do not place your left foot too near your body, otherwise you risk moving further forward than a 90 degree left shin in step 2. Placing your left foot as far as comfortably possible in front of your right knee on the floor is a virtually foolproof way of stretching your upper thigh/hip muscles without causing the tiniest degree of subtle knee damage.

2 Hold onto the support, then, keeping your upper body comfortably upright, and looking straight forward, move forward from the hips toward your left knee as though you were trying to bring the shin of your left leg to a 90 degree angle.

3 Hold the stretch for 30 seconds at your AA, then repeat using the other leg.

calf stretch I

benefits: Tight, inflexible calves can cause lower rear thigh pulls, ankle ligament problems, and painful shin problems. It is therefore important to maintain their full range of motion capability, as muscle fibers are very close together and prone to tightening.

1 Stand with your hands resting just above chest height on a wall, and with your right knee bent and the foot facing forward. Your upper body weight is supported by your arms against the wall, so it does not matter if a slightly acute angle in the knee occurs here.

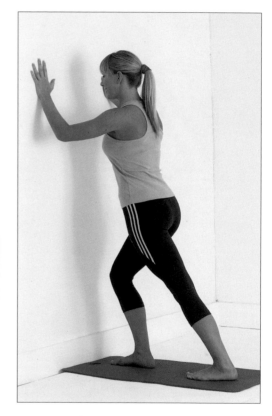

precautions

● Do not allow your left heel to lift off the floor. If it does, you have lost the quality focus of your stretch in that calf and you need to ease back until you feel the AA with the complete underside of the foot in floor contact. This point is vital to the progressive quality of the technique, the result of which should be felt high on the left lower leg.

fact file

● There are two parts to your calf: the curved part that sits on top of the rear leg (the gastrocnemius) and the less prominent but larger and more powerful part that lies beneath it (the soleus). The latter extends from right down at your heel to behind your knee. Both parts require attention if your calves are to be trained properly in flexibility.

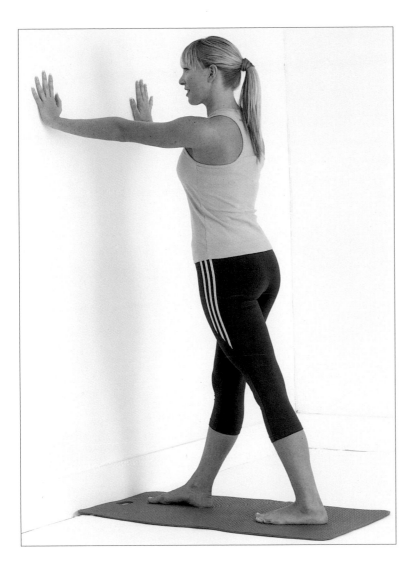

2 Straighten your arms until you are comfortably upright. Now, straighten your left leg out behind you, ensuring you have the entire sole of the foot in contact with the floor.

3 With great care and taking the weight onto your arms as you move, repeat the exercise, bending your right leg a little more and moving forward toward the wall, while still keeping the heel of your left foot constantly in contact with the floor.

4 Hold your AA for 30 seconds, then repeat using the other leg.

calf stretch II

benefits: This stretches the soleus, and the effect will be felt in the Achilles tendon and lower calf.

1 Stand as in step 2 of calf stretch I (see pages 116–117), but with your right foot closer to your left foot and both knees slightly bent.

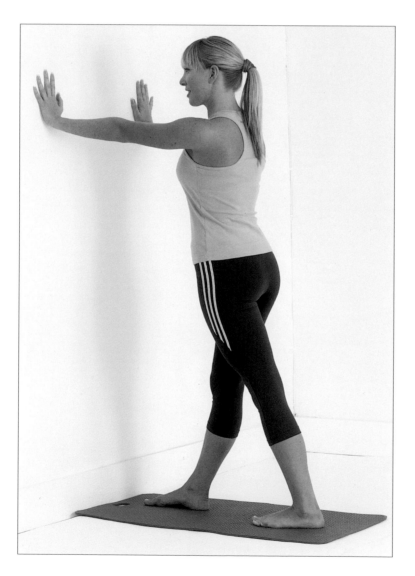

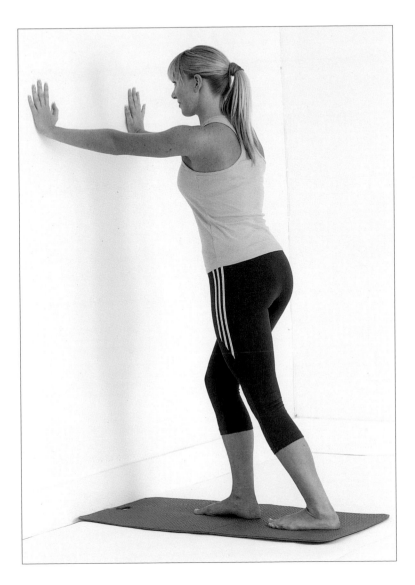

2 Deepen the bend in your right leg
to go forward, as before, but this
time bend the right leg slightly as well
until, as you move slowly forward, you
feel the stretch in the Achilles tendon
and lower calf.

3 Hold your AA for 30 seconds, then
repeat using the other leg.

variation

● As long as your weight is properly
supported against the wall, you can
vary the distance between your front
and back feet and even lower yourself
more at both knees, though avoid
reaching acute angles.

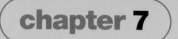

chapter 7

programs

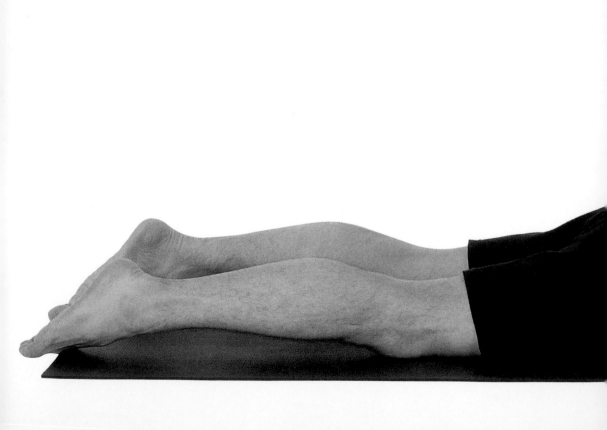

- flexibility for basketball
- flexibility for field hockey and lacrosse
- flexibility for soccer
- flexibility for american football
- flexibility for badminton
- flexibility for volleyball
- flexibility for tennis and squash
- flexibility for backpacking and hiking
- flexibility for long-distance running
- flexibility for middle-distance running
- flexibility for cross-country skiing
- flexibility for cycling
- flexibility for seniors
- flexibility during pregnancy
- "inflight" flexibility

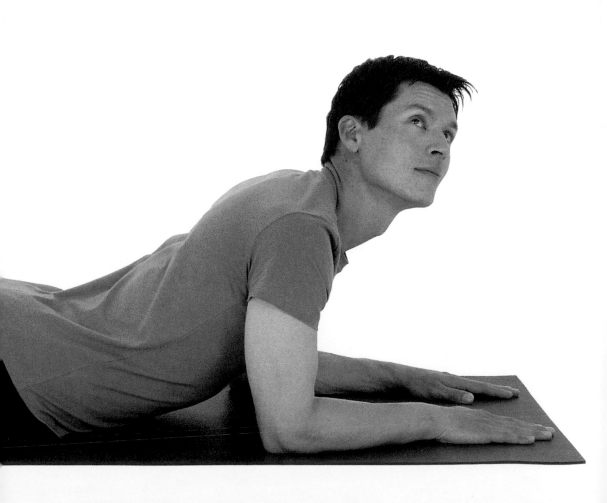

flexibility for basketball

The greatest assets of basketball players are the strength of their legs for the vertical jump and the power of their arms, in particular when they extend their arms in shooting. In addition, the greater height—and therefore the long spinal columns—of the players means that the ability of the lower back to deal with the impact on landing on the court again after jumping for the basket is particularly important.

The importance of the upper back in dealing with the stresses it has to withstand should not be underestimated either. Supporting the arms and shoulders when they are very suddenly required to contract powerfully when either passing or shooting the ball is vital. This is particularly true when the arms are already above the head when the efforts to pass or shoot are made. The higher the arms are away from the center of gravity at the person's midsection, the greater the strength and flexibility in the upper back that is required to make that shot or pass fast and effective without the person pulling a muscle.

Stretching all the areas mentioned is obviously a priority in any player's schedule in order to get a better result all round. Note, however, that, despite the importance of strong legs in basketball, this sport is classified as a direct "torso user." Stretch time will therefore be distributed around the whole body, though with necessarily less time available for multiple leg stretches

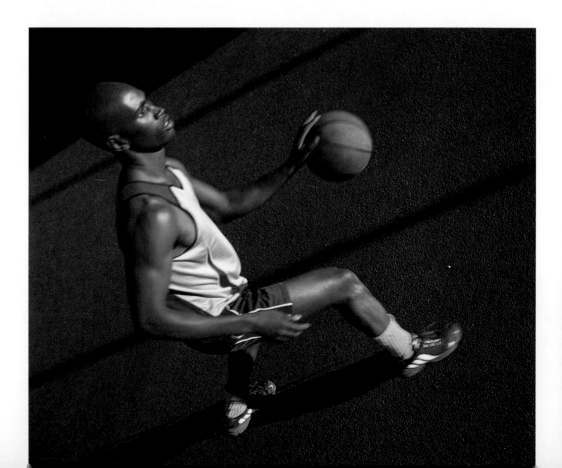

Each of the following stretches should take 60 seconds, except for the standing front thigh stretch, calf stretches, and rear upper arm stretch, where the stretch should be held for 60 seconds on each limb.

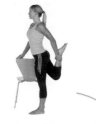

standing front thigh stretch
(see page 105)

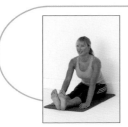

hamstring stretch I
(see page 96)

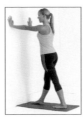

calf stretch I
(see page 116)

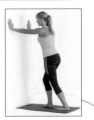

calf stretch II
(see page 118)

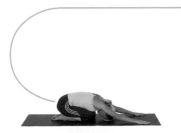

the worshipper
(see page 82)

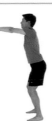

trapezius stretch
(see page 54)

deltoid stretch
(see page 56)

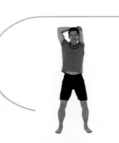

rear upper arm stretch
(see page 52)

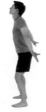

the diver
(see page 44)

cobra stretch
(see page 86)

flexibility for field hockey and lacrosse

The fact that hockey and lacrosse players are holding a stick to their right or left as they play means that their torso will be almost permanently slightly rotated at the waist. This means that there is likely to be an active imbalance in the lower back throughout the game. Such a sustained rotation for long periods can incite possible sciatic nerve problems in the lower back and buttocks (often running down the side of the leg and across the foot), so the buttocks must be included in this stretch routine. The stick itself, though a fairly light burden, is still more than the basic limb weight, and players holding it in front of them and moving it away from the front of their body constantly during play create an increased load for the lower back to balance.

In addition, when hockey and lacrosse players close their grip around the stick, it results in an increased demand on the forearm and wrist muscles. This grip situation can often lead to referred stresses up through to the shoulders, too.

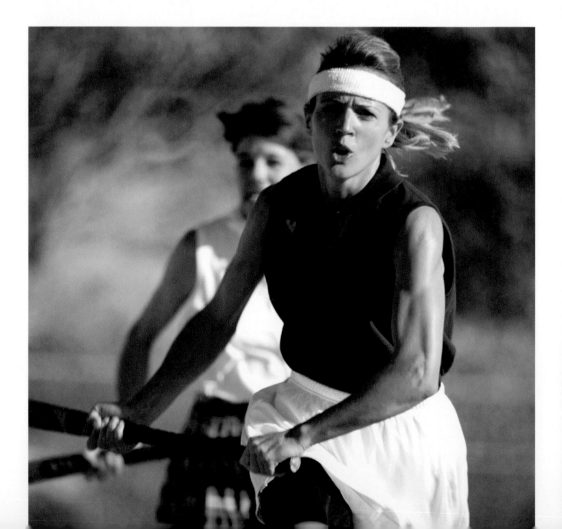

Each of the following stretches should take 60 seconds, except for the hamstring stretch, lying front thigh stretch, knee to chest stretch, calf stretches, gluteal stretch, forearm stretch, and front upper arm stretch, where the stretch should be held for 60 seconds on each limb.

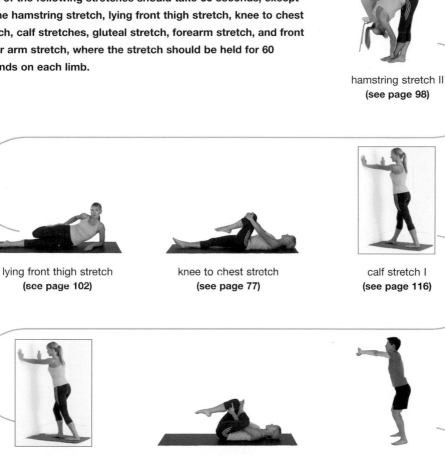

hamstring stretch II
(see page 98)

lying front thigh stretch
(see page 102)

knee to chest stretch
(see page 77)

calf stretch I
(see page 116)

calf stretch II
(see page 118)

gluteal stretch
(see page 111)

trapezius stretch
(see page 54)

the bow
(see page 64)

forearm stretch
(see page 46)

front upper arm stretch
(see page 58)

flexibility for soccer

This sport is a good example of one in which there is a significant biomechanical dominance of the lower body. Soccer players are classified as "non-torso users," because the upper body has no specifically direct involvement in the action. Soccer players, therefore, have the opportunity to devote a little extra time to stretching their lower body, and may place a lower priority (especially if time is short) on attending to the upper body.

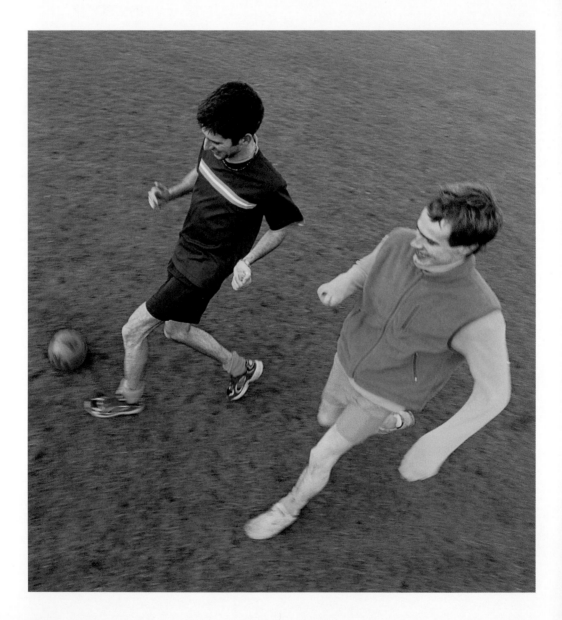

Each of the following stretches should take 60 seconds, except for the lying front thigh stretch, hamstring stretch, inner thigh stretch, calf stretches, gluteal stretch, and ankle stretch, where the stretch should be held for 60 seconds on each leg.

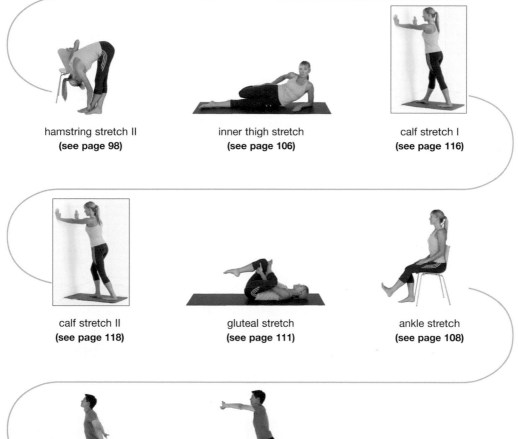

lying front thigh stretch
(see page 102)

hamstring stretch II
(see page 98)

inner thigh stretch
(see page 106)

calf stretch I
(see page 116)

calf stretch II
(see page 118)

gluteal stretch
(see page 111)

ankle stretch
(see page 108)

the diver
(see page 44)

trapezius stretch
(see page 54)

cobra stretch
(see page 86)

flexibility for american football

This sport combines the elements of lower and upper body usage equally, and American football players therefore need to exercise both areas on an equal basis. The extreme physical nature of american football, with its very high levels of impact all over the body, necessitates that the main muscles of postural strength while on the move be attended to in particular. All human postural muscle combinations are less stable when a person is rapidly on the move. To be struck with dramatic force from virtually any direction while moving makes stretching the lower back, stomach, buttocks, and thigh muscles absolutely vital to deliver quality support and protection to the players.

Very few sports, if any, utilize the complete upper body more strenuously than American football, with its raw and consistently violent levels of muscular work in the arms, chest, and shoulders. One of the laws of physiology, which states that "the more you stretch a muscle, the more powerfully it contracts," is highly relevant to American football players, who need to understand that the more powerfully their muscles contract, the greater will be their physical capabilities on the pitch.

The inevitability of dramatically heavy impacts with both opponents and the ground means that highly efficient stretches in all the main large muscle groups of the body are vital. This advice is equally relevant to rugby players.

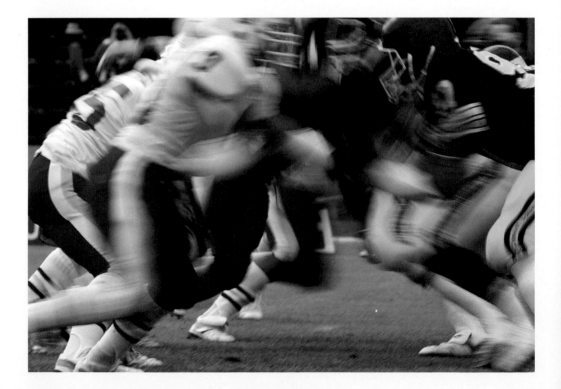

Each of the following stretches should take 60 seconds, except for the standing front thigh stretch and the calf stretch, where the stretch should be held for 60 seconds on each leg.

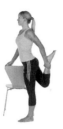

standing front thigh stretch
(see page 104)

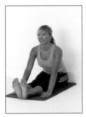

hamstring stretch I
(see page 96)

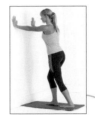

calf stretch II
(see page 118)

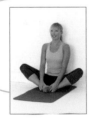

inner thigh stretch
(see page 106)

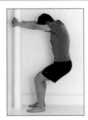

standing lat stretch
(see page 48)

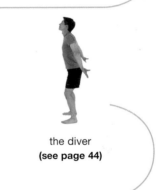

the diver
(see page 44)

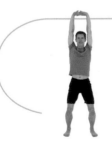

deltoid stretch
(see page 56)

flexibility for badminton

The fact that badminton players are constantly gripping a racket, and favoring one side of their body regarding where they hold it, makes them subject to the same laws as hockey players. The badminton racket is, of course, lighter than the hockey stick, but the badminton player does not have the luxury of being allowed to use both hands to hold it. In addition, the racket will be whirled around rapidly in what often amounts to almost a 360 degree circle.

The eye–hand coordination and reaction times of badminton players are among the fastest around, and the wrist and forearm muscles of their racket arm are under phenomenal split-second stresses during power forehand smashes and whiplike backhand returns.

For any muscular contraction there is a balancing stretch in a partner group without which that contraction could not take place, and this highlights how important good levels of flexibility really are. This very rapid contraction process relating to speed and agility in badminton makes a head-to-toe stretch sequence very important. Badminton players are, by necessity, leaner and lighter in build than hockey players, and strength is very much secondary to agility in this sport.

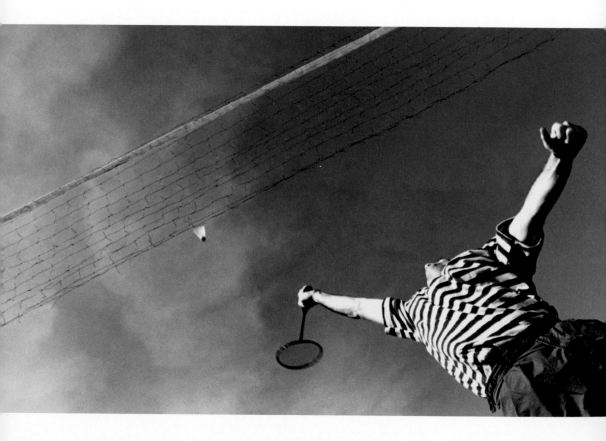

Each of the following stretches should take 60 seconds, except for the lunge stretch, hamstring stretch, calf stretch, rear shoulder stretch, and rear upper arm stretch, where the stretch should be held for 60 seconds on each limb.

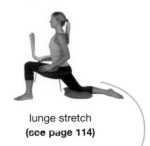

lunge stretch
(see page 114)

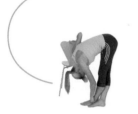

hamstring stretch II
(see page 98)

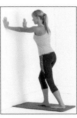

calf stretch II
(see page 118)

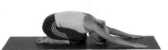

the worshipper
(see page 82)

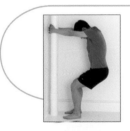

standing lat stretch
(see page 48)

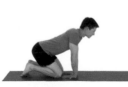

forearm stretch
(see page 46)

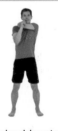

rear shoulder stretch
(see page 50)

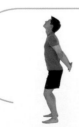

the bow
(see page 64)

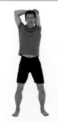

rear upper arm stretch
(see page 52)

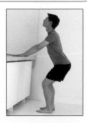

abdominal stretch I
(see page 89)

flexibility for volleyball

Despite the more static nature of volleyball and the lighter ball, biomechanically this sport is very similar to basketball, in that both sports are significantly involved with the ball in the air at arms' length a great deal of the time. This is particularly so in volleyball when players are near the net for a slam situation onto the opponents' court. At these times, body weights are totally off the ground, while the upper body is involved in work that requires it to generate power and speed simultaneously.

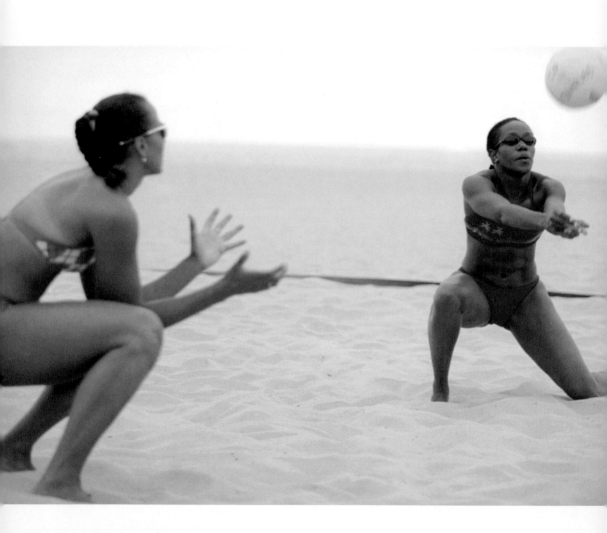

Each of the following stretches should take 60 seconds, except for the standing front thigh stretch, hamstring stretch, calf stretches, and rear upper arm stretch, where the stretch should be held for 60 seconds on each limb.

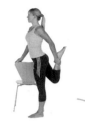

standing front thigh stretch
(see page 104)

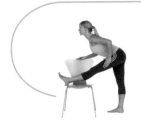

hamstring stretch III
(see page 100)

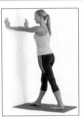

calf stretch I
(see page 116)

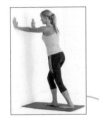

calf stretch II
(see page 118)

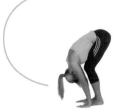

back stretch
(see page 80)

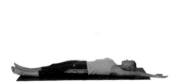

prone and supine hands
(see page 74)

the diver
(see page 44)

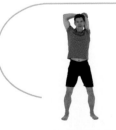

rear upper arm stretch
(see page 52)

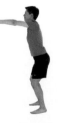

trapezius stretch
(see page 54)

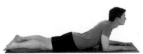

cobra stretch
(see page 86)

flexibility **133**

flexibility for tennis and squash

In human movement terms, squash and tennis are virtually identical, and so in the sport-specific sense the flexibility routine for both is the same. Both are involved with lots of fast sideways, forward, and backward movement, while keeping an eye on the ball. In addition, reaching across the front of the body with the racket arm while on the run, as well as often simultaneously twisting powerfully at the waist, takes place continuously.

In both sports, overhead strokes are as common as sideways ones (and comprise both forehand and backhand techniques), and as the rackets in these disciplines are a little heavier than the badminton one, due consideration to the front upper arm muscle as well as the rear should be given.

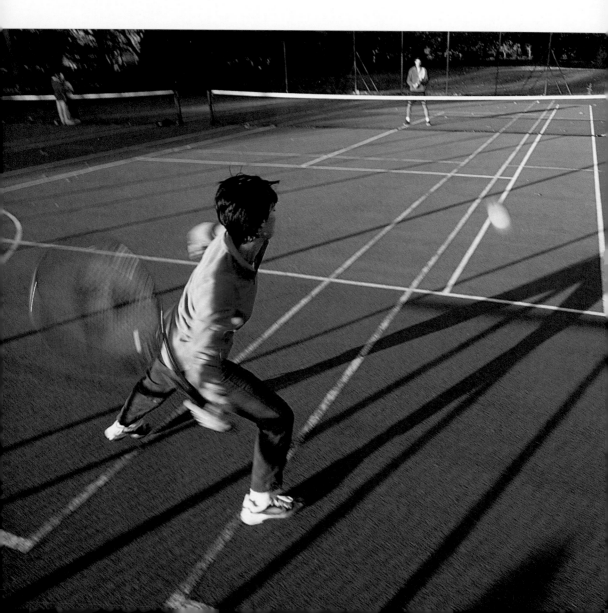

Each of the following stretches should take 60 seconds, except for the standing front thigh stretch, hamstring stretch, calf stretch, rear upper arm stretch, and front upper arm stretch, where the stretch should be held for 60 seconds on each limb.

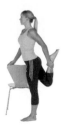

standing front thigh stretch
(see page 104)

hamstring stretch II
(see page 98)

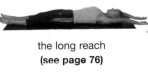

the long reach
(see page 76)

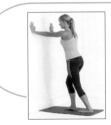

calf stretch II
(see page 118)

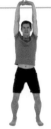

deltoid stretch
(see page 56)

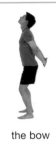

the bow
(see page 64)

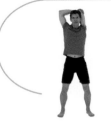

rear upper arm stretch
(see page 52)

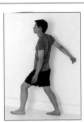

front upper arm stretch
(see page 58)

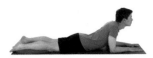

cobra stretch
(see page 86)

flexibility for backpacking and hiking

Both these activities involve walking over what is often rough terrain with what is usually a significant weight on the back, containing tent and outdoor equipment. When the body is weighted and required to move over an uneven surface, the feet and ankles work extra hard in their efforts to keep the body on an even keel. The flexibility and mobility of the ankles are very important here, in order to allow the balance sensors in the feet and ankles to provide the best possible service.

The weight on the back will usually be secured more above the waist than at waist level or below. When loading is placed behind the body's middle to upper back in this way, the work on the lower spinal muscles is particularly demanding even on the flat, never mind ascending a gradient, which can increase the percentage of increased work "awareness" by up to 40 percent. Although the total stresses are borne mainly by the legs, the back muscles make a significant contribution.

The trapezius, combined with the lower spinal muscles, makes the biggest contribution to the strength of the back. Consequently, in terms of a flexibility routine for backpackers and hikers, the greatest attention must be paid to the largest area of the trapezius, along with the lower back and legs.

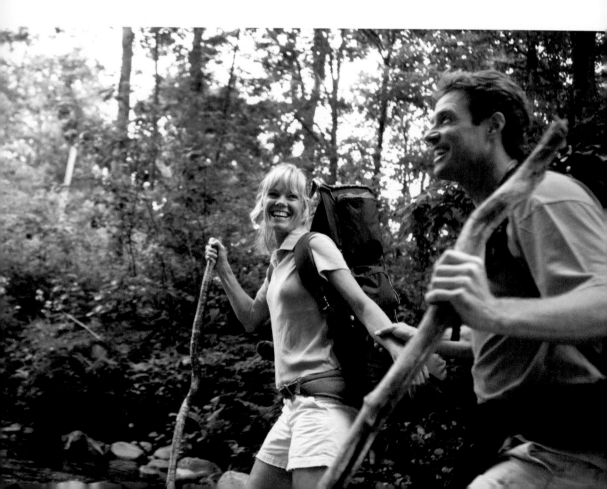

Each of the following stretches should take 60 seconds, except for the standing front thigh stretch, hamstring stretch, knee to chest stretch, rear shoulder stretch, and rear upper arm stretch, where the stretch should be held for 60 seconds on each limb.

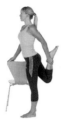

standing front thigh stretch
(see page 104)

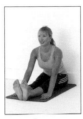

hamstring stretch I
(see page 96)

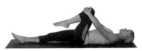

knee to chest stretch
(see page 77)

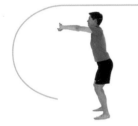

trapezius stretch
(see page 54)

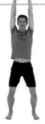

deltoid stretch
(see page 56)

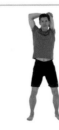

the diver
(see page 44)

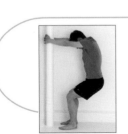

standing lat stretch
(see page 48)

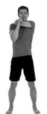

rear shoulder stretch
(see page 50)

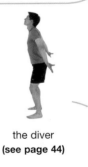

rear upper arm stretch
(see page 52)

flexibility for long-distance running

Although styles in this sport vary, the basic facts are that you must be fairly slim and able to conserve energy to use up carefully as you run. The movement required is a very moderate lift of the leg forward, which uses the upper thighs rather than the lower in order to conserve energy for the mileage to come. A relaxed, energy-conserving arm action is favored. Repeated impact on the lower back and knees, caused by running on what are often roads and other hard surfaces, makes leg flexibility a must for long-distance runners. When these runners run for miles across country, the phenomenal amount of work done by the foot and ankle sensors to keep them from injury is enormous, and so runners must pay good attention to their ankles. For this reason, 60 seconds should be allocated to stretches concerning the lower back, legs, calves, and ankles, as they bear the full brunt of the loading.

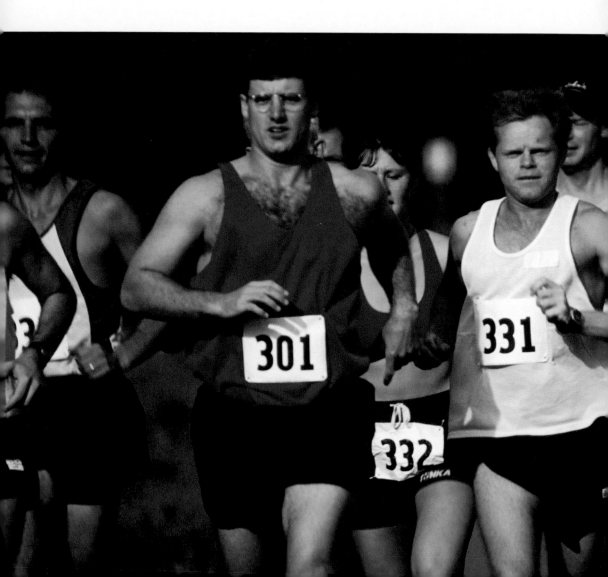

Each of the following stretches should take 60 seconds, except for the lunge stretch, hamstring stretch, calf stretches, and ankle stretch, where the stretch should be held for 60 seconds on each leg.

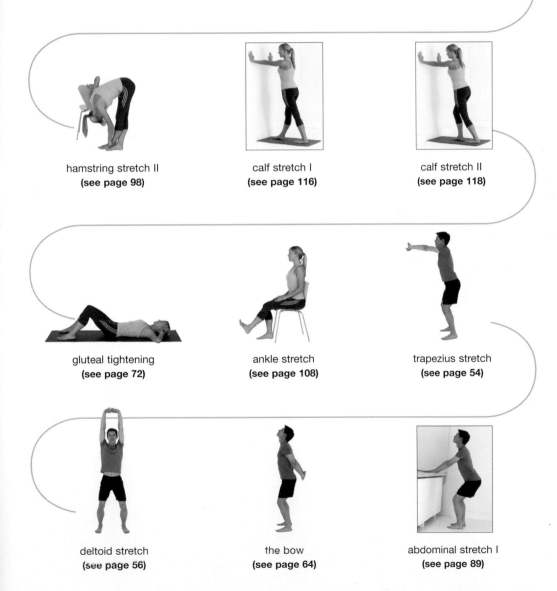

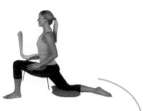

lunge stretch
(see page 114)

hamstring stretch II
(see page 98)

calf stretch I
(see page 116)

calf stretch II
(see page 118)

gluteal tightening
(see page 72)

ankle stretch
(see page 108)

trapezius stretch
(see page 54)

deltoid stretch
(see page 56)

the bow
(see page 64)

abdominal stretch I
(see page 89)

flexibility for middle-distance running

Middle-distance runners and sprinters need to accelerate rapidly and expend energy at a much quicker rate than long-distance runners, in order to travel faster over the shorter distances involved. The leg lift is therefore much higher and the driving-down force of the leg is much more dynamic and makes increased use of the lower part of the front upper thigh muscle near the knee.

The power-oriented nature of middle-distance running means that runners need powerful "piston" arm contributions to their efforts to drive themselves forward at greater speed. These differences make them "torso users" despite the fact that no racket, bat, or other implement is used, except in relay races with a baton. Their arms are fairly flexed and tensed in the dynamics of this technique, making them instrumental to the success of runners' endeavors. A full-body approach is therefore needed for such runners.

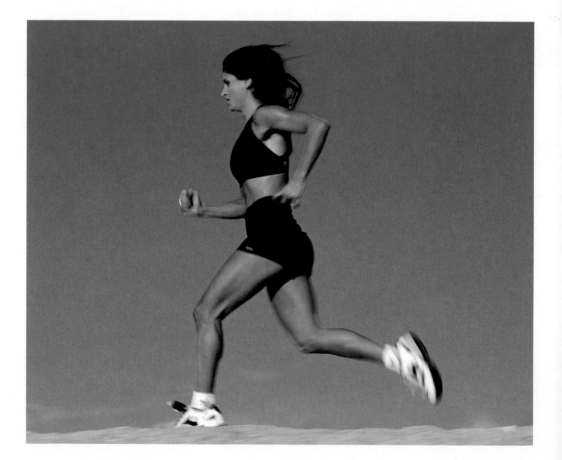

Each of the following stretches should take 60 seconds, except for the standing front thigh stretch, hamstring stretch, knee to chest stretch, rear upper arm stretch, and front upper arm stretch, where the stretch should be held for 60 seconds on each limb.

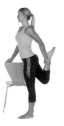

standing front thigh stretch
(see page 104)

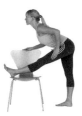

hamstring stretch III
(see page 100)

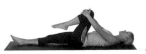

knee to chest stretch
(see page 77)

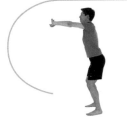

trapezius stretch
(see page 54)

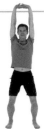

deltoid stretch
(see page 56)

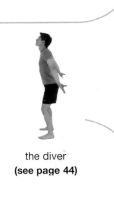

the diver
(see page 44)

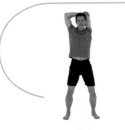

rear upper arm stretch
(see page 52)

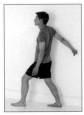

front upper arm stretch
(see page 58)

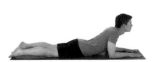

cobra stretch
(see page 88)

flexibility for cross-country skiing

This sport is probably one of the most all-round demanding single-activity sports in existence. Skiers have to negotiate gradients over long distances in snow, and sliding and lifting the legs forward over and over, while using both arms independently to provide assistance, is a very demanding biomechanical process. The legs are not able to drive the body forward as intended because the surface of the snow creates an energy-sapping medium that allows much less traction than the legs are seeking. The arms are then recruited to drive the ski sticks down and back in an attempt to assist matters, which places considerable workloads on the chest, rear upper arms, and upper back, so making this a "torso user" type of sport. As two sticks/implements are involved, they constitute two separate individual units being used independently through at least 180 degrees of movement on either side of the body. This requires even more effort and control to maintain successfully.

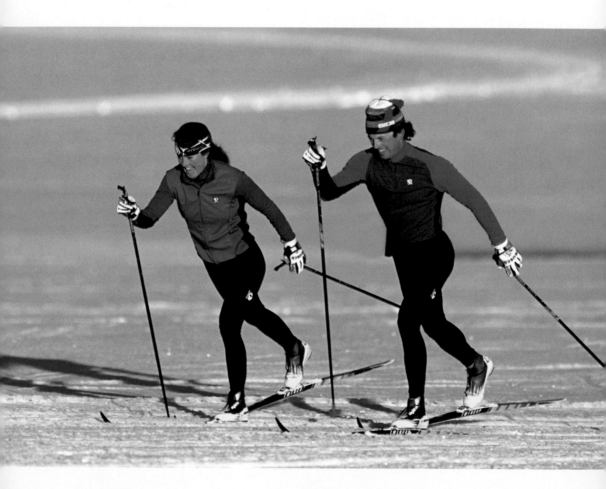

Each of the following stretches should take 60 seconds, except for the lying front thigh stretch, hamstring stretch, rear upper arm stretch, front upper arm stretch, and ankle stretch, where the stretch should be held for 60 seconds on each limb.

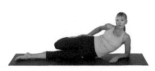

lying front thigh stretch
(see page 102)

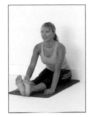

hamstring stretch I
(see page 96)

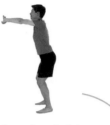

trapezius stretch
(see page 54)

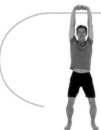

deltoid stretch
(see page 56)

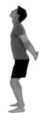

the bow
(see page 64)

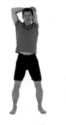

rear upper arm stretch
(see page 52)

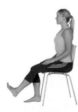

front upper arm stretch
(see page 58)

ankle stretch
(see page 108)

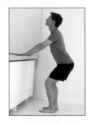

abdominal stretch I
(see page 89)

flexibility for cycling

This is obviously one of the most leg-oriented activities there is, and so cyclists need a good leg flexibility routine. In order to gain a significant training effect from cycling, it is generally agreed that 9.4 mph needs to be maintained. This means that most cyclists tax their legs long and hard, so stretches for the front lower and upper thigh muscles must be included, as their efficient teamwork is the foundation of the cyclist's success or failure.

Other muscles that need to be attended to are the buttocks, which can become sore, and the wrists, which suffer from having the muscles on top of the forearm locked in one position when holding the handlebars for too long. The inner thigh/groin area must also be attended to, including the rear upper arm muscles, which endure long periods of being used with the arms in a half-flexed position. This can place a heavy load, particularly on the part of those muscles nearest the elbows.

Each of the following stretches should take 60 seconds, except for the lunge stretch, standing front thigh stretch, hamstring stretches, calf stretch, knee to chest stretch, rear shoulder stretch, and rear upper arm stretch, where the stretch should be held for 60 seconds on each limb.

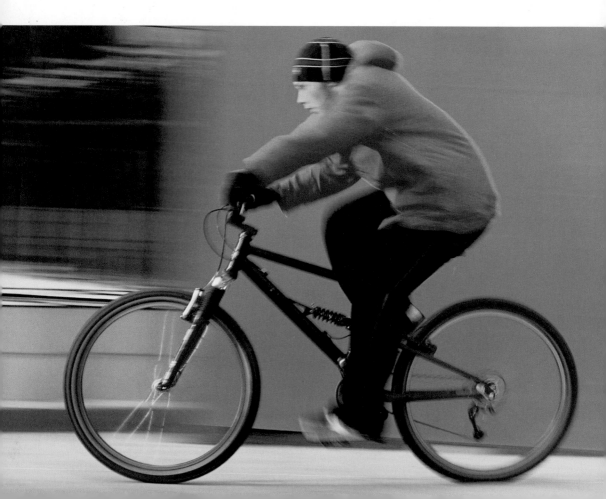

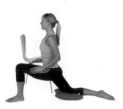

lunge stretch
(see page 114)

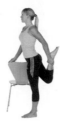

standing front thigh stretch
(see page 104)

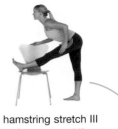

hamstring stretch III
(see page 100)

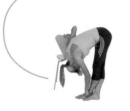

hamstring stretch II
(see page 98)

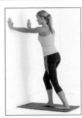

calf stretch II
(see page 118)

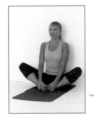

inner thigh stretch
(see page 106)

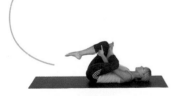

gluteal stretch
(see page 111)

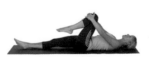

knee to chest stretch
(see page 77)

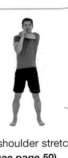

rear shoulder stretch
(see page 50)

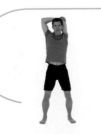

rear upper arm stretch
(see page 52)

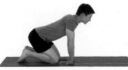

forearm stretch
(see page 46)

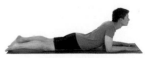

cobra stretch
(see page 86)

flexibility for seniors

The benefits of flexibility for older people are resoundingly obvious: it improves their quality of life through better mobility and greater ranges of comfortable motion. Improving people's flexibility automatically improves their ability to perform tasks in simple daily life that would otherwise be an irritating nuisance. Simply bending down without effort or turning quickly in reacting to a situation without suffering from a back twinge for the rest of the day (or longer)—these are bonuses that are well worth getting.

Suitable stretches are those that are solid and safe, and if those exercises listed here are performed regularly within the principles and guidelines of this book, they will expand and enhance physical capabilities to a pleasing and significant degree.

Each of the following stretches should take 60 seconds, except for the hamstring stretch, lying front thigh stretch, ankle stretch, calf stretch, and rear upper arm stretch, where the stretch should be held for 60 seconds on each limb.

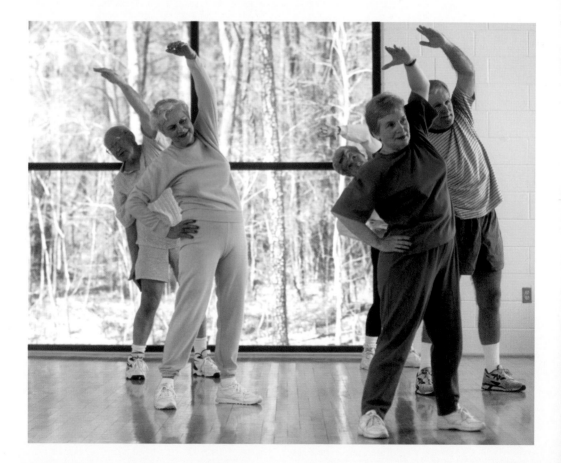

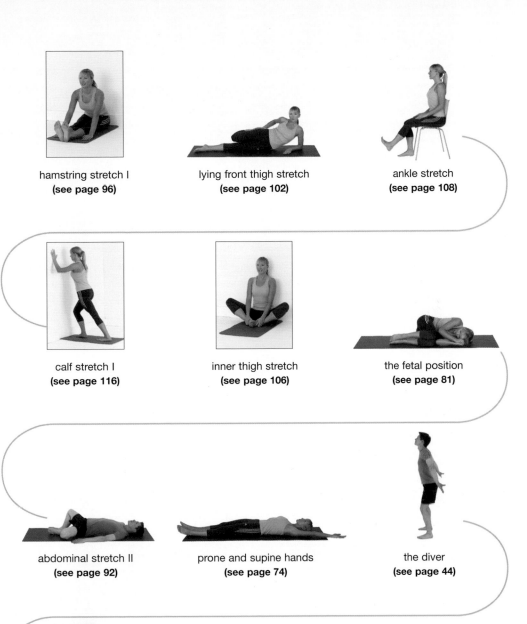

hamstring stretch I
(see page 96)

lying front thigh stretch
(see page 102)

ankle stretch
(see page 108)

calf stretch I
(see page 116)

inner thigh stretch
(see page 106)

the fetal position
(see page 81)

abdominal stretch II
(see page 92)

prone and supine hands
(see page 74)

the diver
(see page 44)

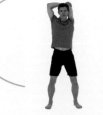

rear upper arm stretch
(see page 52)

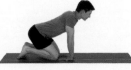

forearm stretch
(see page 46)

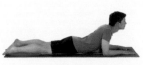

cobra stretch
(see page 86)

flexibility during pregnancy

The most important aspects of stretches suitable for expectant mothers are their gentleness and the lack of risk of sustaining any significantly uncomfortable muscular contractions in the lower back, or compressing the abdominal area in any significant way. Each pregnancy is, however, unique, with its own individual circumstances, and although the stretches listed opposite are suitable for anything up to seven and a half months, pregnant women should always check with their physician or consultant before embarking on a stretch routine, however safe and gentle.

Spinal disc and/or associated bladder nuisances can be a relevant factor in your training. For example, if you are suffering from pressures on either of these areas while pregnant, listen to your body and choose only stretches that feel comfortable. Labile blood pressure (fluctuating blood pressure) scenarios, which are often common during pregnancy, are helped by the soothing and relaxing medium of gentle stretching.

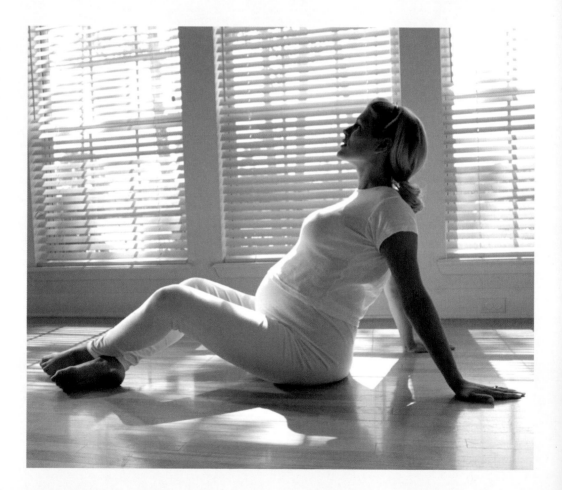

Each of the following stretches should take 60 seconds, except for the lying front thigh stretch and hamstring stretch, where the stretch should be held for 60 seconds on each leg.

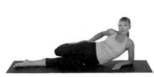

lying front thigh stretch
(see page 102)

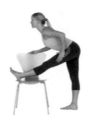

hamstring stretch III
(see page 100)

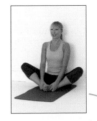

inner thigh stretch
(see page 106)

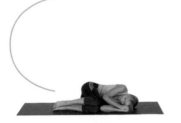

the fetal position
(see page 81)

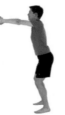

trapezius stretch
(see page 54)

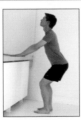

the diver
(see page 44)

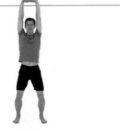

deltoid stretch
(see page 56)

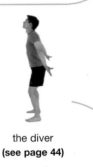

abdominal stretch I
(see page 89)

"inflight" flexibility

Flying has always been a period of near-to-total immobility, and long-haul flights in particular cause even very fit people to become stiff after sitting or half lying for extended hours at a time.

The space around seats is never generous enough to enable fliers to perform full head-to-toe programs, but a little gentle stretching can be easily (and fairly discreetly) achieved, and this is all that is needed to arrive at a destination feeling relatively alert and fit. By tilting their seats back a little, fliers can perform the following exercises simply by adapting them to the seated rather than the standing position.

Much has been said about DVT (Deep Vein Thrombosis) being a danger associated with air travel, particularly on long haul flights. Despite the often alarmist nature of the information provided, it has not been clinically proven that this is a condition associated in isolation with air travel. DVT occurrences have claimed older, sedentary, unfit individuals whose static lifestyles were probably an influential factor. So don't be static on these flights. Stretch, keep the blood flowing more efficiently, and create your own insurance policy against such conditions.

By tilting your seat back a little and simply sitting instead of assuming a standing posture, you will be able to accomplish:
- Seated shoulder stretch, arms straight forward, palms facing away from you.
- Ankle rotations.
- Seated, drooping down forward from the waist between your legs, lower back stretch.

In the toilet for 30 seconds each:
- Foot on seat, rear upper thigh, stretch.
- Standing left hand to right foot, front upper thigh stretch.
- Seated, arms straight and directly above the head, palms away from you, shoulder stretch.
- Standing, stomach stretch, palms on a ledge.
- Standing chest stretch, arms straight behind back, hands at buttock level.

This would be enough to loosen you up nicely, but make sure you lock the door!

Each of the following stretches should take 60 seconds, except for the ankle stretch, hamstring stretch, and standing front thigh stretch, where the stretch should be held for 60 seconds on each leg.

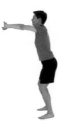

trapezius stretch
(see page 54)

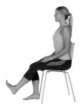

ankle stretch
(see page 108)

back stretch
(see page 80)

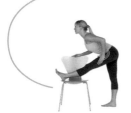

hamstring stretch III
(see page 100)

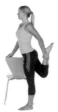

standing front thigh stretch
(see page 104)

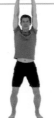

deltoid stretch (seated)
(see page 56)

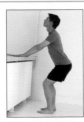

abdominal stretch I
(see page 89)

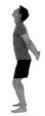

the bow
(see page 64)

resources

fitness organizations

American Alliance for Health, Physical Education, Recreation, & Dance
1900 Association Dr.
Reston, VA 20191-1598
TEL: 703-476-3400
WEB SITE: www.aahperd.org

IDEA Health & Fitness Association
10455 Pacific Center Court
San Diego, CA 92121-4339
TEL: 800-999-4332, ext. 7
FAX: 858-535-8234
WEB SITE: www.ideafit.com
E-MAIL: contact@ideafit.com

Australian Fitness Network
Suite 2, 25 Grosvenor Street
Neutral Bay, NSW 2089
TEL: 02 9908 4944
FAX: 02 9908 4349
WEB SITE: www.fitnessnetwork.com.au
E-MAIL: info@fitnessnetwork.com.au

books

Total Stretch
Roscoe Nash
MQ Publications, 2003
A progressive program suitable for beginner and intermediate levels detailing body specific stretches accompanied by step-by-step photography.

Relax Into Stretch: Instant Flexibility Through Mastering Muscle Tension
Pavel Tsatsouline
Dragon Door Publications, 2001
An illustrated guide to the 36 most effective techniques for increasing your flexibility.

Stretching: 20th Anniversary (Stretching, 20th Ed.)
Bob Anderson
Shelter Publications, 2000
An easy-to-use book on stretching for all age groups and fitness levels.

Fit For Life
Ranulph Fiennes
Little, Brown and Company, 1999
This book by the man known as "the world's greatest living explorer" provides useful advice that is eminently suitable for both beginners and intermediate exercisers.

useful Web sites

www.bhfactive.org.uk
The British Heart Foundation Web site has advice on exercise, nutrition, and living a healthy lifestyle.

www.exercise.co.uk
Healthy food recommendations, training tips, and alternative treatments to aid your well-being.

www.fitness-training.net
Detailed discussion of stretching techniques and flexibility.

www.gssiweb.org
The Gatorade Sports Science Institute Web site is very well put together and appealing to all levels of visitor.

www.healthyliving.gov.uk
Useful information about healthy nutrition and physical activity.

www.hfonline.co.uk
News about health and fitness. The mind and body section links to yoga tutorials.

www.howtostretch.com
Detailed instructions on how to stretch your body, with accompanying photos.

www.marathontraining.com
General stretching advice and its benefits and importance for runners.

www.mayoclinic.com
Helpful medical and practical advice on stretching.

www.netfit.co.uk
A selection of exercises, fully illustrated.

www.nutrition.org.uk
The British Nutrition Foundation Web site is a very good discloser of extensive nutritional information.

www.patient.co.uk
A very comprehensive health promoting and active lifestyle site.

www.personalhealthzone.com
Articles and links on health, fitness, weight loss, and nutrition.

www.prevention.com
US health and fitness magazine with a really versatile content.

www.sportsinjurybulletin.com
Stretching and flexibility tips to help avoid sports injury and radically improve overall athletic performance.

www.webhealthcentre.com
Safe guide to stretching exercises.

www.wholefitness.com
Some simple stretching suggestions for warming-up, cooling-down, and relieving harmful stress.

glossary

AA point The "annoying ache" point is the name given to the stage when you begin to feel a mild sensation of resistance and tension in a target muscle when you gently stretch it. The point where you can feel the effect of a stretch on your body.

Achilles tendon The strong tendon that joins the muscles in the calf of the leg to the heel bone. It is the thickest and strongest tendon in the human body.

Abdominals (abs, rectus abdominis) These stomach muscles are made up of many different sections. Abdominal muscle consists of a thin layer of muscle that starts from the base of the breastbone and runs down to the pubic bone area.

Abduction, abductor Abduction is movement *away* from the center of the body. An abductor is a muscle whose contraction results in this movement.

Adduction, adductor Adduction is movement *toward* the center of the body. An adductor is a muscle whose contraction results in this movement.

Articulation The joint or connection between two or more bones or cartilages in a skeleton.

Ballistic stretching A method of stretching that is slowly being eliminated owing to the danger of uncontrolled bouncing movements acting as a trigger to the stretch reflex (a part of the muscle that increases muscular tension to avoid any tearing within the muscle). It is also sometimes known as bounce stretching.

Belly (of a muscle) This is the name given to the fleshy center of a muscle.

Bicep (biceps brachii) A large two-headed muscle at the front of the upper arm that bends the forearm toward the shoulders. The biceps function in pulling and curling movements.

Biomechanics This is the science derived from studying all the components of the human musculo-skeletal sysyem in motion.

Calories Used to describe the energy value of nutrients. Calorie beginning with a capital "C" is the common term for kilocalorie (kcal), while calorie with a lowercase "c" is one thousandth of a kilocalorie.

Calves The muscles at the back of the lower leg. Their main function is to allow you to raise your heel for walking and running, etc.

Circulation The flow of blood through the body's blood vessels caused by the pumping of the heart. Stretching is very beneficial to the circulation.

Cool-down A series of slow, stretching exercises performed after a more strenuous activity or training session, which help to remove waste products from the body and helps the heart rate return to normal.

Core This refers to the lower back and abdominal muscles. The core is themost important area for stabilizing the body during movement and it is involved in every twitch, contraction, and movement you make.

Deltoid (delt, musculus deltoideus)
A large three-part muscle (front, side, and rear deltoid) of the shoulder that moves the arms away from the body.

Dehydration A condition resulting from the excessive loss of body water. It can lead to fainting, nausea, and vomiting, which unfortunately further escalates the condition.

Eu-stress This is the name for the positive kind of stress that you thrive on and which motivates you to continue working.

Flow A strength-training term referring to smooth, continuous movements from exercise to exercise without any interruption in focus.

Focus A mental process used when training to concentrate on the exercise and the muscle that you are working.

Gastrocnemius The main calf muscle, giving the calf its strong, rounded shape. Despite providing the visible curved profile to the rear lower leg, this muscle is actually the smallest of the two major muscles there. It is stretched and exercised most efficiently with the leg in a straight position.

Glute (gluteus maximus, buttock, bottom, rear) The outermost muscle of the three glutei found in each of the human buttocks and the strongest muscle in the human body.

Hamstring (ham, biceps femoris, posterior thigh muscle) Any of the three muscles at the back of the thigh that function, to flex and rotate the leg and extend the thigh.

Intercostals The muscles that lie between the ribs.

Intervertebral discs The pads of tissue found between the vertebrae (the bones of the spinal column). They act as cushions between the vertebrae, protecting the spine from everyday stress.

Inverse myotatic reflex This safely stops the momentum of the myotatic reflex, preventing the muscle from being stretched beyond its maximum length and damaged.

Isolation This refers to exercising or stretching one specific muscle exclusively, without the involvement of any other muscles.

Kyphosis The abnormal backward arching or curvature of the spine, producing a hunchback appearance often accompanied by round shoulders.

Lats (latissimus dorsi) The fan-shaped muscles that flare out to either side of the upper torso.

Ligaments Straplike structures consisting of dense, fibrous tissue, which are positioned in such a way as to allow movement, but also to restrict the range of movement to within a safe level to prevent damage to adjacent tissues and structures.

Lumbar spine The lower five vertebrae of the spine commonly referred to as the small of the back. This is the strongest part of the spine, which provides structural support for the body.

Metabolic rate The rate at which the body converts energy stores in the form of calories into working energy in a given period of time.

Muscles Each muscle in the body has a main part and two ends—the tendons. Muscles are usually attached on the two bones on either side of a joint via their tendons, and when the main part contracts, it shortens.

Muscular contraction The shortening and thickening, or tensing, of a muscle or muscle fiber.

Myelin sheath An insulating fatty layer that covers and protects the nerve fibers in the body.

Myotatic reflex This allows a muscle to stretch out completely unhindered. However, this reflex is unsafe because once a muscle goes beyond its maximum length, it can tear.

Pace This term refers to the speed at which you train and it will vary according to personality, fitness, mood, and various other external factors.

Pectorals (pecs, musculus pectoralis) The two broad fan-shaped muscles across the chest. Their prime function is abducting the arms—moving the arms across the chest—as well as assisting in the movement of the shoulder and upper arm.

Personal trainer An advanced exercise and nutrition professional, whose clinical training is measured in years, not weeks or months, and whose experience measures at least 5–8 years after this level of training. He or she will teach, motivate, and inspire you, working one-on-one with you to help you develop a suitable personalized training routine.

Physiology The biological study of the vital functions and processes of living organisms—cells, tissues, organs, etc.

Prone hands When the hands are palms down in a stretch position.

Quadricep (quad, musculus quadriceps femoris) A major four-part muscle in the front thigh primarily engaged in extending the leg at the knee.

Repetition or rep One complete movement of an exercise.

Rhomboids These are the muscles in the upper back. They help to move the shoulder blade.

Rotator cuff A structure around the shoulder joint that is made up of muscles and tendons that stabalize the shoulder.

Routine The sum of reps, sets, and exercises in any given workout.

Sciatic nerve The largest nerve in the body. It runs from the lower back down to the lower limbs providing sensory and motor function to the lower extremities.

Scoliosis This is a pronounced sideways tilt or curve to the spine, which can lead to chronic back problems. It can be caused when one side of the back is less flexible than the other.

Set The prescribed number of repetitions of any given exercise. Example: one set of eight repetitions.

Soleus Flatter than the gastrocnemius, but larger in size, this muscle extends from underneath the gastrocnemius behind the knee and tapers down over a greater length of the rear lower leg to the heel. It is exercised and stretched most efficently with the leg bent.

Spasm An involuntary and abnormal muscular contraction.

Static stretching This involves holding a stretch at a point where the muscle is under full stretch.

Supine hands When the hands are palms up in a stretch position.

Tendon A band of strong and fibrous (collagenous) tissue, often cordlike in appearance, which connects muscles to bones and other structures.

Torso This refers to the muscles in your trunk and midsection: abdominals, obliques, erectors, and intercostals.

Tricep (tri, triceps brachii) A large horseshoe-shaped, three-headed muscle on the back of the upper arm. It is used primarily for extending the elbow, thus straightening the arm.

Thermoregulation The process by which the body maintains its internal temperature within a certain tolerable range despite a varying environmental temperature.

Trapezius (traps) A large flat triangular muscle that goes into the base of the skull and spreads across the shoulders on both sides of the neck and down the upper back. It is involved in moving the shoulders and arms and is often responsible for tension headaches.

Vertebrae The individual bones that make up the spinal column and support the back. There are 33 in the human body.

Warm-up A series of gentle movements and exercises performed before a training session or strenuous activity to prepare the muscles and joints, increase heart rate and circulation, and encourage concentration.

Workout A collection of exercises, usually performed either at the gym or in your home. Also used to describe one complete exercise session.

index

Entries in *italics* refer to names of stretches